Easy Embryology
Dr Minass

First published in 2021.

Hardback: 978-0-6485925-5-6
Paperback: 978-0-6485925-7-0
eBook: 978-0-6485925-4-9

All inquiries should be made directly to the author by e-mail at m.inass@outlook.com.

Content and illustrations by Dr. Minass.

Preface

No longer will the words "embryology" and "confused" be used in the same sentence. This book is dedicated to the simplification of embryology.

Essentially, embryology is the process of turning two cells, a sperm and an egg, into a human baby. Every organ in your body develops from a bunch of cells that will evolve to reach their final functional form. Embryology explains how this process occurs.

Two things to note prior to turning the page. First, as a first-year student learning embryology, you'll probably be asked to learn the development of an organ before you even know what embryology is. However, understanding the embryology of specific organs is dependent on first understanding the process of fertilisation to gastrulation. This is because every organ is derived from the trilaminar disc resulting from gastrulation (ectoderm, mesoderm, and endoderm). Therefore, it would be wise to first understand this process prior to learning about the development of individual systems.

Second, the aim of this book is to keep embryology simple. As a result, only normal development is described in this book. As well as avoiding the anomalies, the molecular regulation of organ development is also omitted in this book for the same reason. Anomalies and clinical scenarios will be included in Easy Embryology: Part 2.

Chapter 1: Before the Beginning

Before the oocyte and the sperm cell, there were primordial germ cells (PGC). The PGC do not appear in the embryo until week two, but they are responsible for the development of the oocyte and the sperm cell. A cellular "what came first, the chicken or the egg?" scenario.

1.1 Primordial Germ Cells

From the second to the seventh week of gestation, the PGC travel from the epiblast through the primitive streak to the continually developing gonads via the yolk sac. During this five-to-six-week journey, they continue to divide by a process called mitosis (Image 1.1).

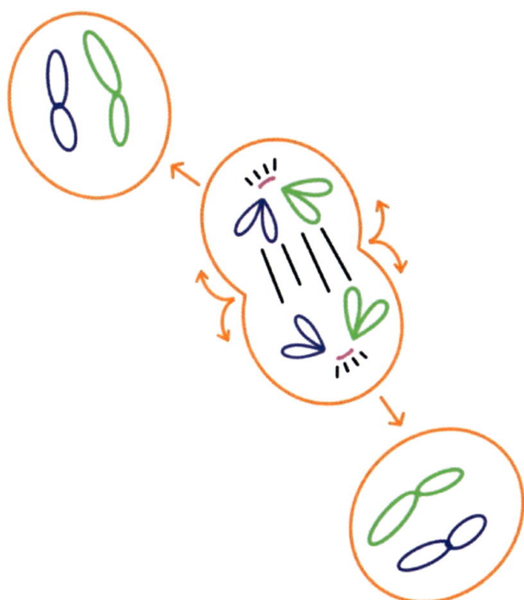

Image 1.1: Mitosis.

1.2 Oogenesis

Oogenesis is the development of a mature oocyte from a PGC in the ovary. When the PGCs arrive, they differentiate into oogonia. Ongoing mitosis of the oogonia results in the appearance of many more oogonia and by week 12 each cluster of oogonia is surrounded by follicular cells.

Most of the oogonia continue to undergo mitosis but some of them 'freeze' at meiosis I and become primary oocytes (Image 1.2).

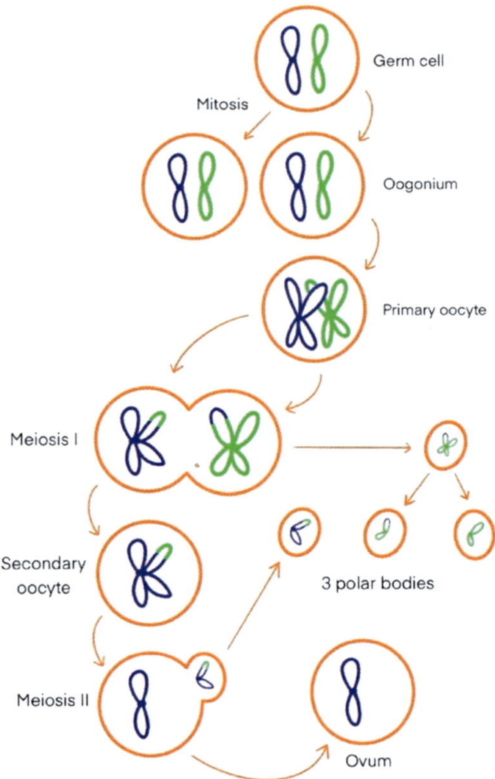

Image 1.2: Maturation of the oocyte.

A primary oocyte surrounded by follicular cells is called a primordial follicle. All primary oocytes remain frozen in meiosis I until puberty. Image 1.2 paired these similar sounding words with the relevant cell for your understanding.

During meiosis, the original cell divides into four, but only one will become a mature oocyte. The other three cells are the polar cells. Polar cells barely have any cytoplasm and they end up dying, but that one mature oocyte that survives and undergoes meiosis II has 23 chromosomes (one of which is the X chromosome).

High Yield!

The cells involved in oogenesis appear in the following order:

1. PGC
2. Oogonia
3. Primary oocyte (inside a primordial follicle)
4. Growing oocyte (inside a secondary follicle)
5. Secondary oocyte (inside a graafian follicle)
6. Mature oocyte (ovum).

At puberty for females, every month around 20 cells mature into the antral phase, then they mature into the graafian follicle right before ovulation. The follicular cells become granulosa cells, and the thecal cells develop to produce steroids. In each cycle, only one oocyte reaches maturity while the others die. Prior to ovulation, meiosis I completes but remains frozen in meiosis II. Meiosis II will only complete if the oocyte gets fertilised with a sperm.

1.3 Ovarian cycle

If you're a medical student or doctor, then you MUST know the ovarian cycle. Not just for embryology, but because knowing the ovarian cycle is important for clinical reasoning and diagnosis in obstetrics and gynaecology. Taking the history is the most important part of making any diagnosis.

High Yield!

The effects of oestrogen include:

- Endometrial proliferation and cervical mucus thinning which makes the environment more "hospitable" for sperm
- Inhibition of the Hypothalamus-Pituitary-Gonadal (HPG) axis when released in small amounts – this is how the contraceptive pill works, by preventing ovulation and
- Augmenting of the HPG axis by provoking a surge in luteinising hormone (LH) and follicle stimulating hormone (FSH) when oestrogen is released in higher amounts.

The LH surge at midcycle has the effect of:

- Stimulating progesterone production and
- Causing follicle rupture and ovulation.

The ovarian cycle in a textbook-healthy female is a regular monthly cycle that begins at puberty. The hypothalamus is the all-seeing all-knowing control centre of this cycle. Specifically, the HPG axis is in charge. Simply put the hypothalamus releases gonadotropin releasing hormone

(GnRH) which stimulates the anterior pituitary gland to release LH and FSH.

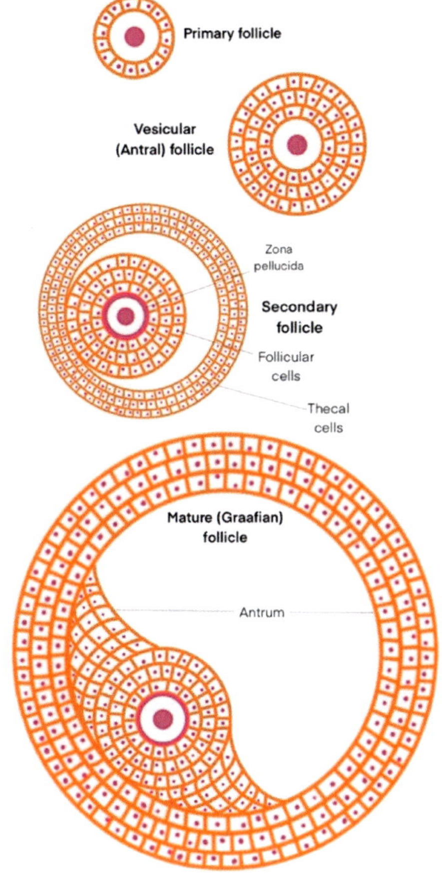

Image 1.3: Oogenesis.

LH pushes thecal cells to make steroids such as androstenedione, and FSH makes the granulosa cells convert androstenedione to oestrogen. Initially, only a little bit of oestrogen is being produced. At this low concentration oestrogen inhibits the HPG axis. However, as the follicle grows and the granulosa cells are producing more and more oestrogen, it has the opposite effect, triggering the HPG axis. In essence, a surge of LH from thecal cells causes the follicle to rupture, releasing the oocyte. This is called ovulation. The follicle now becomes the corpus luteum and secretes progesterone. If fertilisation doesn't occur, the corpus luteum degenerates into the corpus albicans. The corpus albicans is a chunk of scar tissue that no longer makes progesterone. This is represented in Image 1.4.

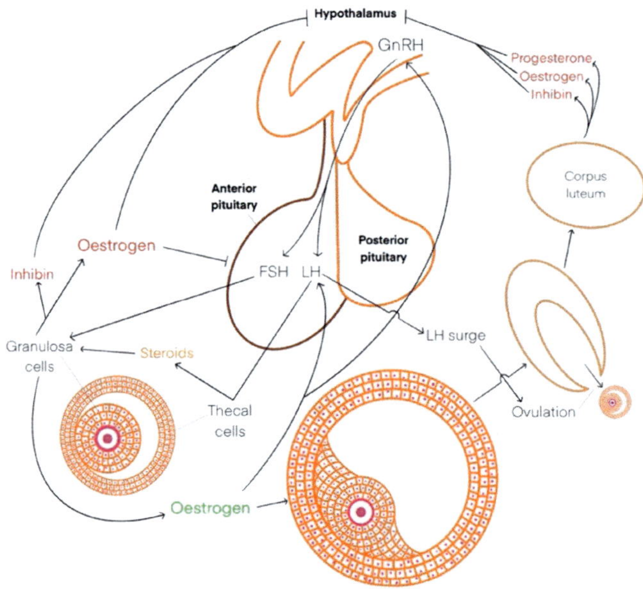

Image 1.4: The HPG axis and the ovarian cycle.

1.4 Spermatogenesis

Spermatogenesis begins at puberty for males and is regulated by the HPG axis (Image 1.5). In this situation, LH tells the Leydig cells to stimulate the production of testosterone, and FSH stimulates the Sertoli cells to guide spermatogenesis by producing androgen binding protein.

Sertoli cells protect the developing sperm cells and provides them sustenance as they mature.

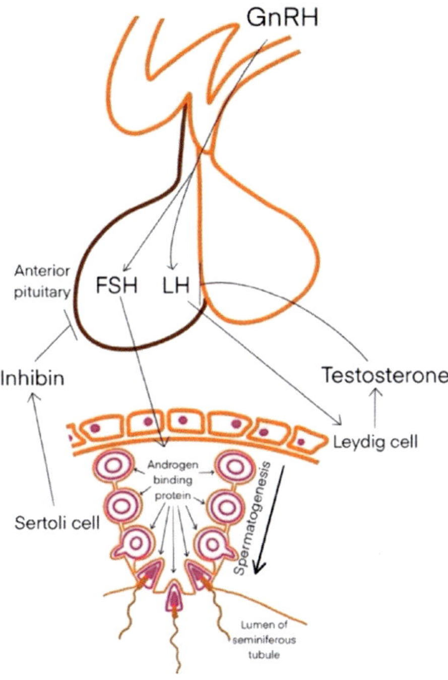

Image 1.5: The HPG axis that regulates testosterone production and spermatogenesis.

The PGCs in males differentiate into stem cells that give rise to type A spermatogonia. Mitosis of these cells produces type B spermatogonia which divide further into primary spermatocytes, secondary spermatocytes, and finally into spermatids. Image 1.6 shows the hierarchy of sperm. Throughout each division, the developing sperm cell is joined by life-sustaining cytoplasmic bridges. Without this life-sustaining bridge, sperm development ceases.

1.5 Spermiogenesis

Spermiogenesis is the process of spermatids becoming spermatozoa. First, an acrosome is formed which contains ingredients that arm sperm with the ability to invade an oocyte during fertilisation. Then the nucleus condenses, and the neck, middle piece, and tail are formed. At this point the cytoplasm is no longer needed and is therefore discarded. When mature, spermatozoa enter the seminiferous tubules and are moved toward the epididymis by a motion similar to peristalsis (similar to how the oocyte travels down the uterine tube following ovulation). Once in the epididymis, sperm should be Olympic-level swimmers.

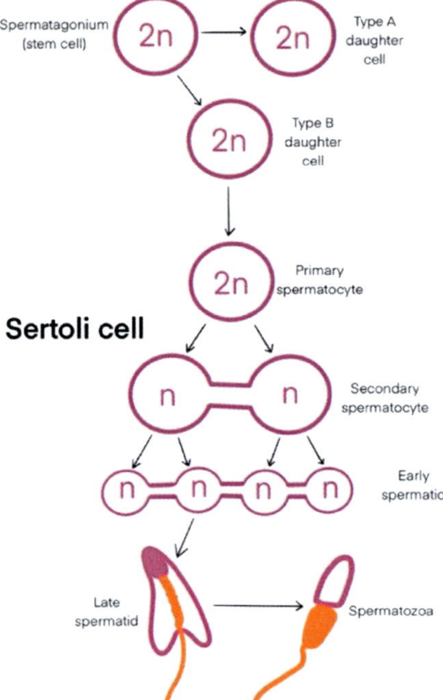

Image 1.6: Spermatogenesis (and spermiogenesis).

Chapter 2: Fertilisation to Gastrulation

This is arguably the most important chapter in the book. To understand any other aspect of systems-based embryology, a good understanding of the process of fertilisation to gastrulation is needed. The result of gastrulation yields a three-layer germ disc which is the genesis of every other thing that will be discussed from Chapter 3 onward.

2.1 Fertilisation

Fertilisation is the process of the sperm and oocyte fusing together to form a zygote. This usually occurs in the ampulla of the uterine tube. Only 1% of sperm that was lucky enough to make it inside the vagina makes it into cervix. From the top 1% that make it in the uterus, only a fraction is pushed up into the uterine tubes by the uterus with its muscular contractions. Contrary to popular belief that all movement of sperm is due to their impeccable athletic ability, only a small amount of their movement is contributed by "swimming".

Sperm fertilise the egg by first undergoing capacitation by losing their glycoprotein coating and their seminal plasma proteins. Without this step, sperm cannot undergo the next step, the acrosomal reaction. The acrosomal reaction is simply a reaction involving the acrosome, where enzymes, like acrosin, in the sperm are released that help it penetrate the zona pellucida like in Image 2.1.

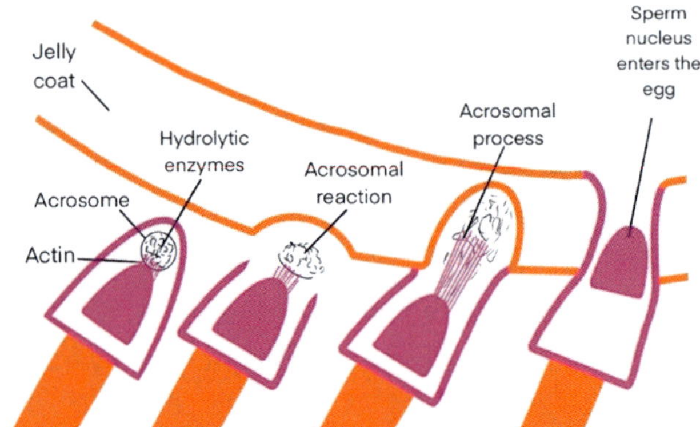

Image 2.1: Fertilisation.

High Yield!

The phases of fertilisation are:

1. Corona radiata is penetrated
2. Zona pellucida is penetrated and
3. Zona pellucida induces the zona reaction.

When sperm enters the oocyte, the cortical and zona reactions prevent any more sperm entering and the second meiotic division continues. Resulting from fertilisation, the diploid number of chromosomes are restored (23 from oocyte and 23 from sperm) and the sex of the new future baby is determined too (XX or XY).

2.2 Cleavage

Following fertilisation, cleavage occurs. Cleavage is the word for when the zygote undergoes many mitotic divisions as demonstrated in Image 2.2.

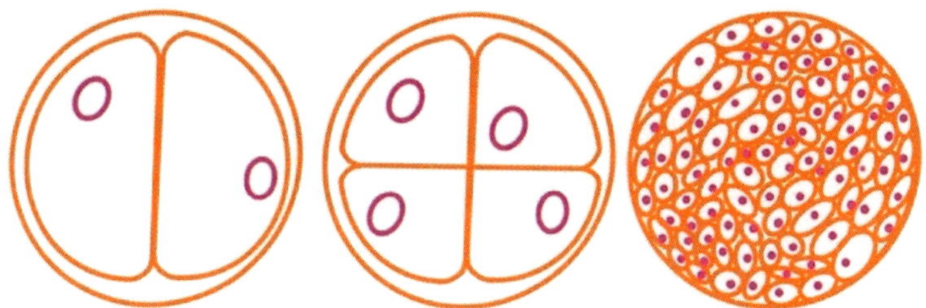

Image 2.2: This is what happens following fertilisation. The fused egg and sperm divide becoming a solid ball of cells by the time it reaches the lumen of the uterus (day 3-4). Left: The first division. Centre: Another division. Right: A solid ball of cells.

2.3 Implantation

A 16-cell-strong ball is known as the morula. The morula has an inner cell mass and an outer cell mass. The inner cell mass gives rise to the embryo and the outer cell mass forms the trophoblast. When fluid enters the morula and creates a cavity, the ball of cells is now known as the blastula. The blastula is the entity that will implant into the endometrium. This journey is summarised in Image 2.3 and 2.4.

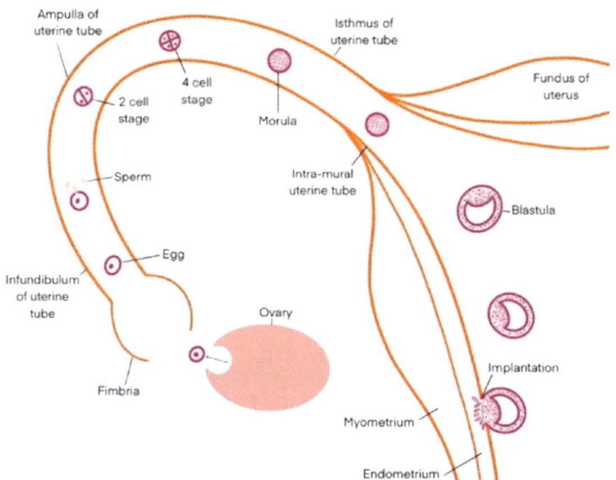

Image 2.3: The events from ovulation to implantation.

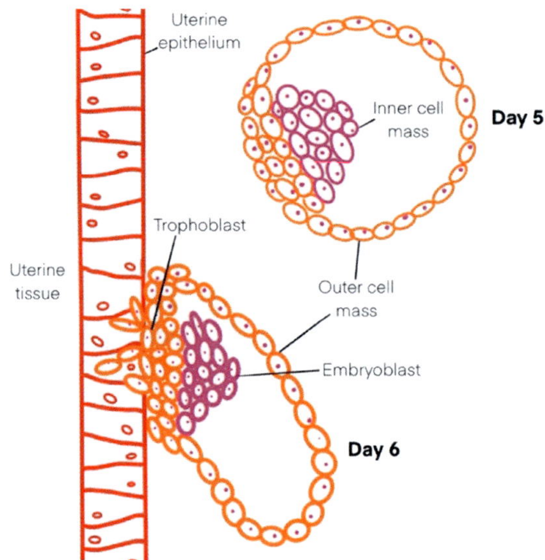

Image 2.4: Implantation.

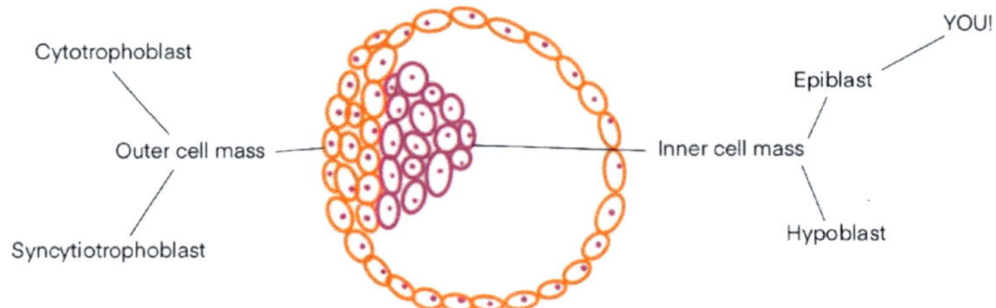

Image 2.5: You are an epiblast.

On day nine, the trophoblast forms lacunae, and in two days the lacunae expand to form a system of cavities connected. Just think of the lacunae as empty spaces that are at first only holes, but then some of the holes join with other holes to form a tunnel system. This tunnel system will become the foetal circulation! Eventually maternal blood enters the network and the uteroplacental circulation commences (Image 2.6).

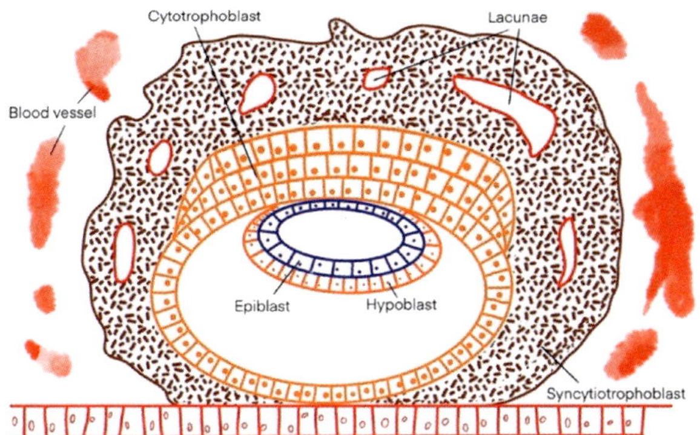

Image 2.6: Day 9.

In week three, the trophoblast has primary villi. Mesodermal cells enter these villi forming secondary villi, and they differentiate to become blood cells and blood vessels. This forms a circulatory system, and the secondary villi are now known as the tertiary villi. All that is needed now is a pumping baby heart to get the blood flowing.

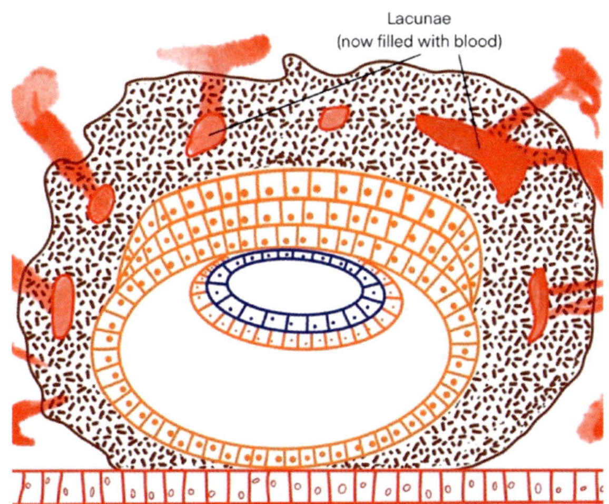

Image 2.7: By day 12 maternal blood enters the lacunae as they are now a network. Note that by day 12 there is more differentiation between each embryoblast than is shown in this image.

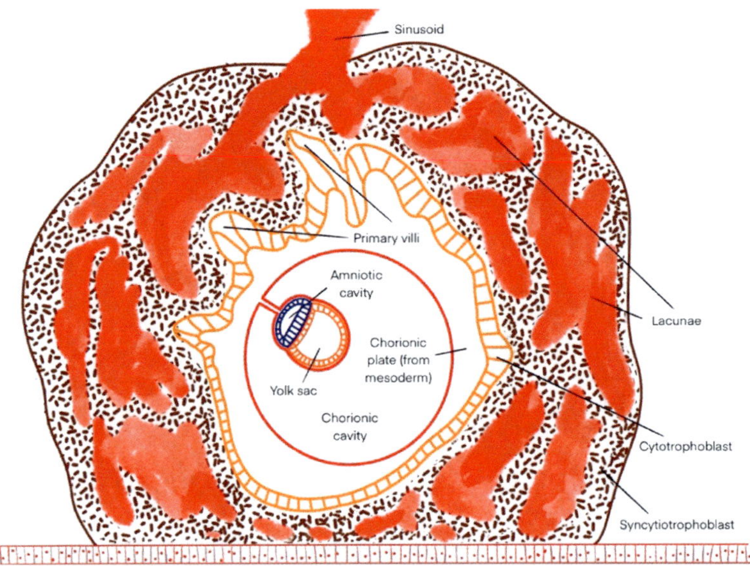

Image 2.8: The uteroplacental circulation on day 13. Primary villi are the fingers of the cytotrophoblast that encroach into the syncytiotrophoblast.

2.4 The Placenta

The placenta is created from the trophoblast and the chorionic plate (which is extraembryonic mesoderm). Maternal blood arrives to the placenta from the uterine spiral arteries. These arteries disintegrate, willingly, to release blood which bathes the villi. The villi invade the ends of the spiral arteries like a Chinese finger trap, and this is how the circulation is established.

The placenta continues to grow to keep up with the increasing metabolic demands of the foetus. The function of the placenta is to exchange metabolic and gas products between mother and foetus, and to produce hormones.

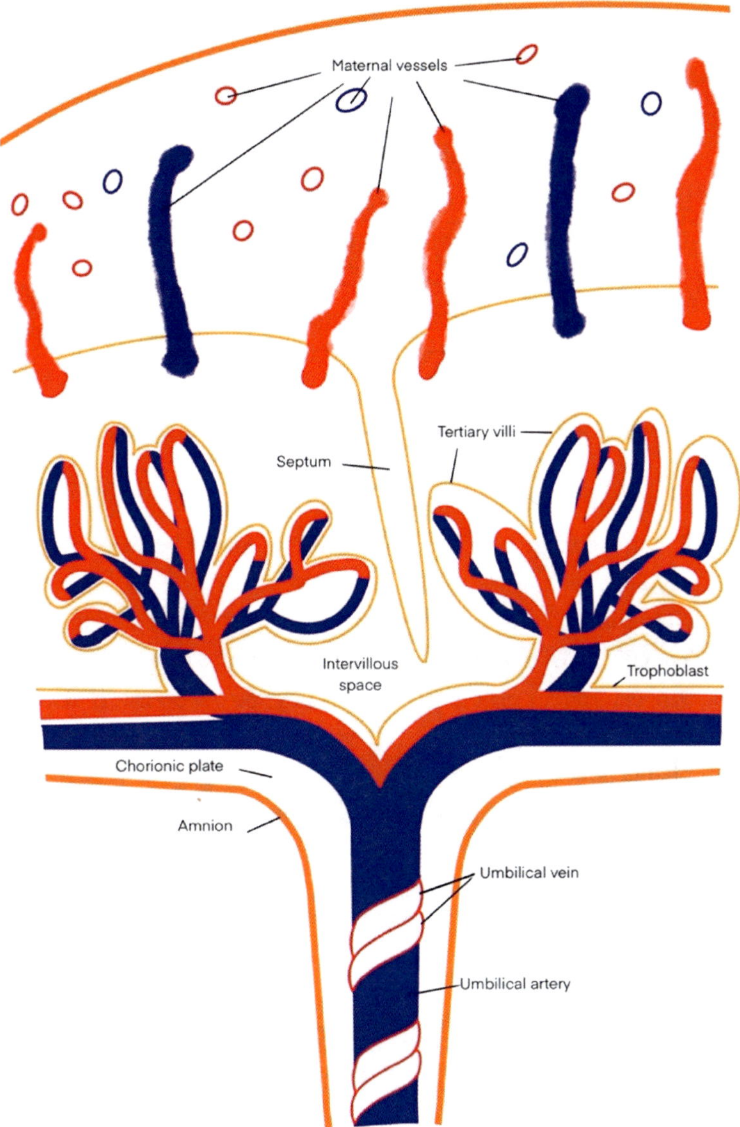

Image 2.9: Uteroplacental circulation.

High Yield!

The blood flow through the placenta is summarised as follows:

- Blood is received from up to 100 spiral arteries from mama
- This blood pushes its way into the spaces between villi covering each villus in oxygenated blood
- When the pressure from mama's blood decreases, the blood flows back entering the endometrial veins and
- There is a membrane in the placenta, fittingly called the placental membrane, that separates foetal and maternal blood.

The functions of the placenta are:

- A fair exchange of oxygen and carbon dioxide between mama and baby
- Nutrients and electrolyte exchange between mama and baby
- Transferral of antibodies (IgG only) from mama to baby
- Progesterone is produced by the syncytiotrophoblast. It also produces oestrogens which helps the uterus and mammary glands develop and
- The syncytiotrophoblast produces human chorionic gonadotropin which maintains the corpus luteum.

2.5 Gastrulation

From the epiblast come the three germ layers, and by the third week they finally appear. These layers are the **ectoderm** (outer layer), **mesoderm** (middle layer), and **endoderm** (inner layer). The process of development of these three layers is called gastrulation. Initially though, they seem more like the upper, middle, and lower layer since they start out as three flat layers like a stack of pancakes.

When the primitive streak is formed on the epiblast, gastrulation begins. Cells of the epiblast move towards the middle where the streak is and enter it (Image 2.10). Once the cells enter, they push the hypoblast out of the way so that the invading epiblast cells can become the endoderm. More cells enter through the primitive streak and lay between the new endoderm and the epiblast forming the mesoderm. The rest of the epiblast becomes the ectoderm.

A common misconception is that the hypoblast becomes the endoderm. This isn't true as the ectoderm, mesoderm and endoderm all come from the epiblast. That is, the epiblast is the source of everything that becomes you (ectoderm, mesoderm, and endoderm). See Image 2.5: You are an epiblast.

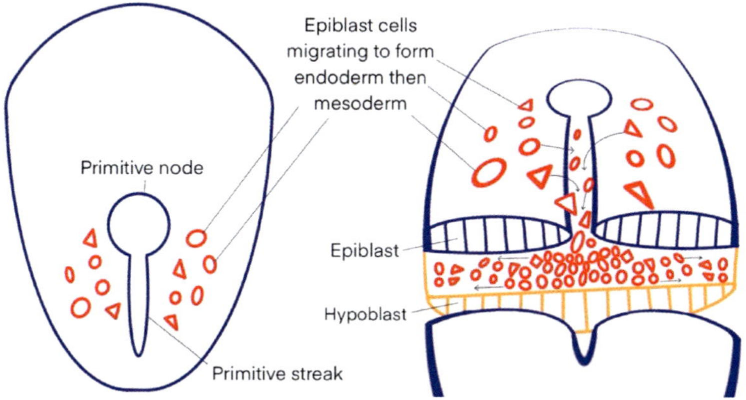

Image 2.10: Left: view of the embryoblast from the top. Right: cross-sectional view of the "pancake" (don't write pancake for your exams, the proper term is embryoblast). The epiblast cells push the hypoblast to form the endoderm and mesoderm.

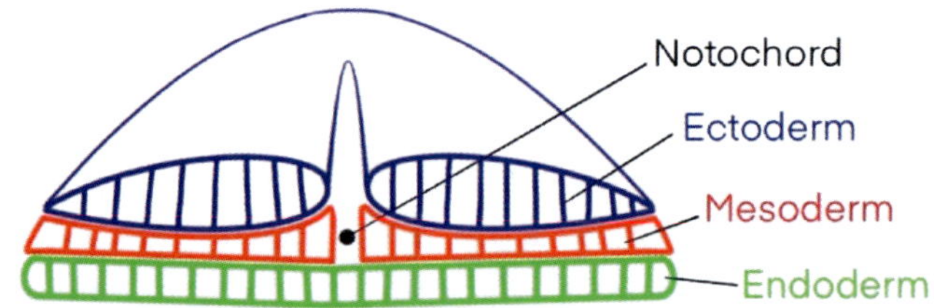

Image 2.11: Day 18: the three germ layers.

2.6 The Notochord

The notochord is a long pole that runs down the midline of the embryoblast. It is made from cells that make up the axis in which the future vertebrae are assembled around. It is the foundation of the axial skeleton and is first noticeable around day 13. There are three stages to notochord development, these are: the notochordal process stage, the pre-chordal stage, and the notochordal stage.

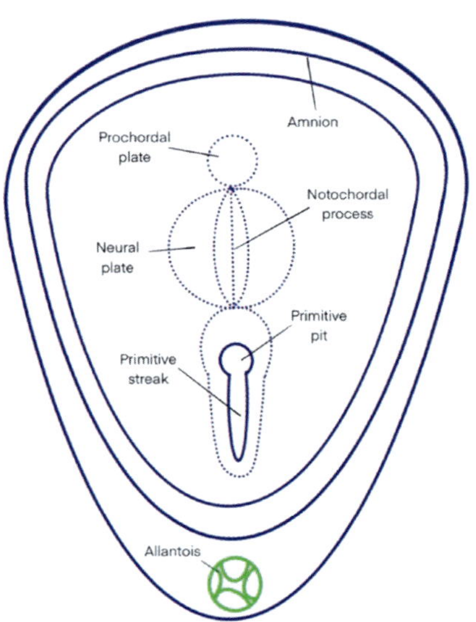

Image 2.12: Looking at the embryo (when it is in the flat disc "pancake" stage) from the top at around day 18. The pro-chordal plate is endoderm.

2.6.1 The Notochordal Process Stage

Pre-notochordal cells enter the primitive streak with one mission: to make it to the pro-chordal plate, which is a mere slab of thickened endoderm. This extends all the way up from the primitive streak. In this stage, the developing notochord is still attached to endoderm.

2.6.2 Pro-chordal stage

As the endoderm is being formed during gastrulation, the notochordal cells multiply and pinch off the hypoblast. The fused region is no more and new lumens form. Now the yolk sac, the notochordal canal, and the amniotic cavity are connected by an open passageway as shown in Image 2.13.

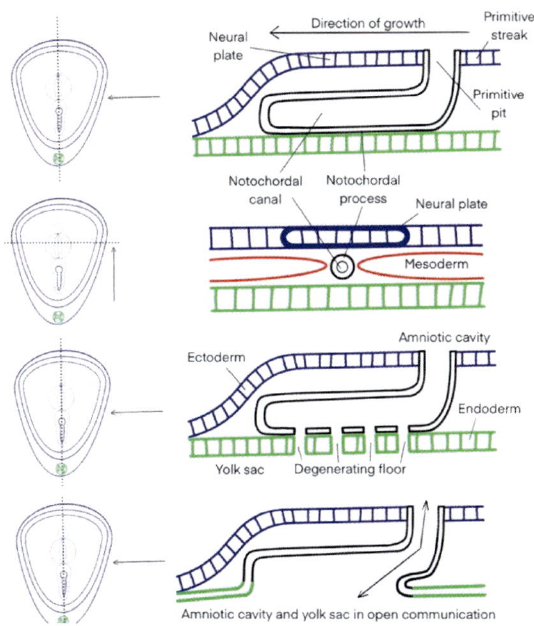

Image 2.13: Pro-chordal stage.

2.6.3 Notochord stage

The notochordal process becomes a plate which folds into itself to form a cord. The folding begins at the top end all the way down to the bottom. The holes in the endoderm are filled and there is no longer an open communication linking the yolk sac to the amniotic cavity. The notochord is now a single solid cord of cells which sits underneath the neural tube.

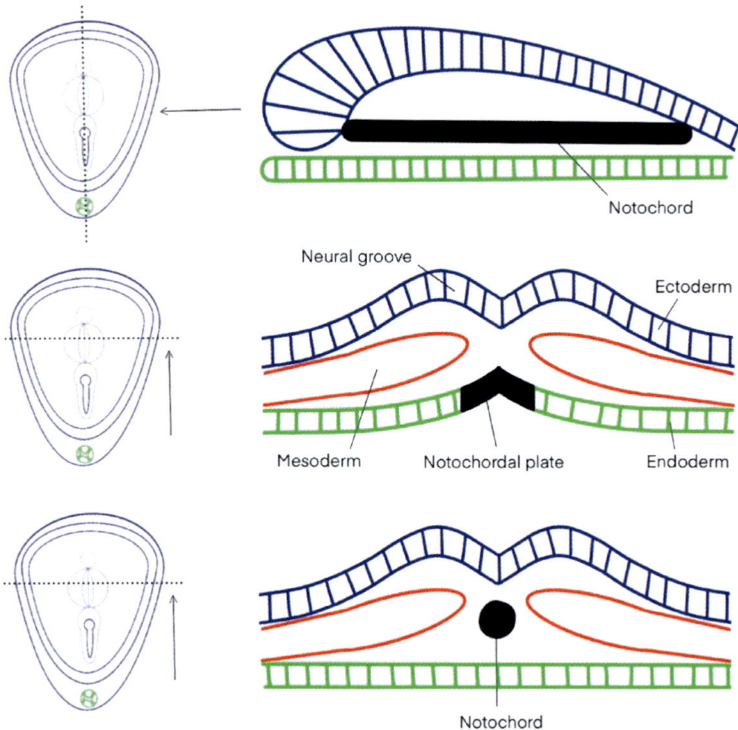

Image 2.14: Notochord stage. The notochord is developed by day 19.

2.7 Neurulation

Neurulation is the process of the neural tube "pinching off" the ectoderm to form the beginning of the Central Nervous System (CNS). While it is connected to the ectoderm it is known as the neural plate.

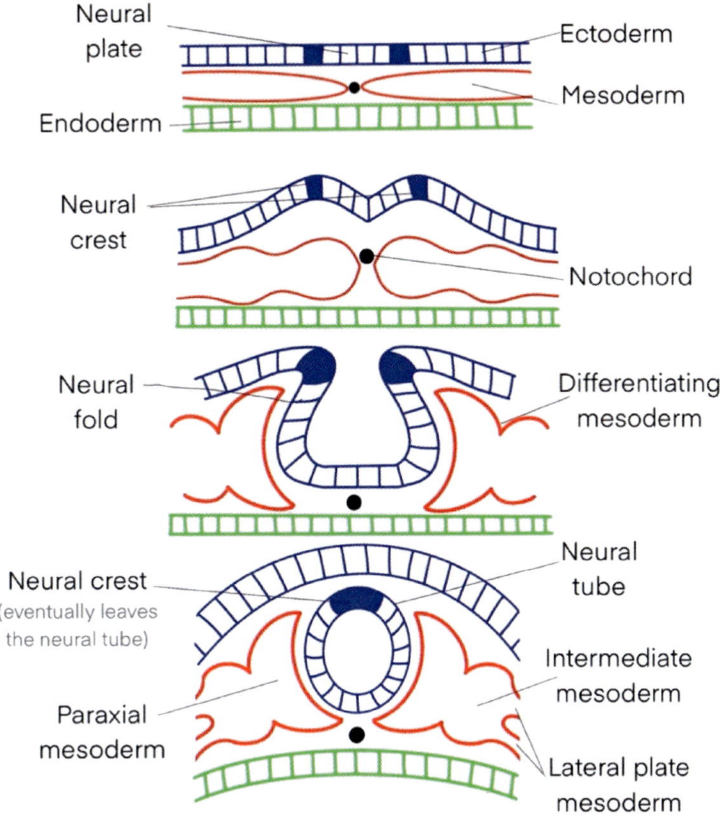

Image 2.15: Neurulation. The neural plate pinches off the ectoderm forming a tube. It is much easier to visualise what occurs in this cross-section view than it is from a dorsal view.

Around day 21, the two furthest ends of the neural plate fold up to become the neural folds. Once both ends meet and come off the ectoderm, it is known as the neural tube (check out Image 2.15).

The top end of the neural tube is open and is called the anterior neuropore. The bottom end is also open and is called the posterior neuropore. Failure of closure of the anterior or posterior neuropore leads to abnormalities (anencephaly and spina bifida respectively). Neurulation is complete when they close, and what remains is the CNS.

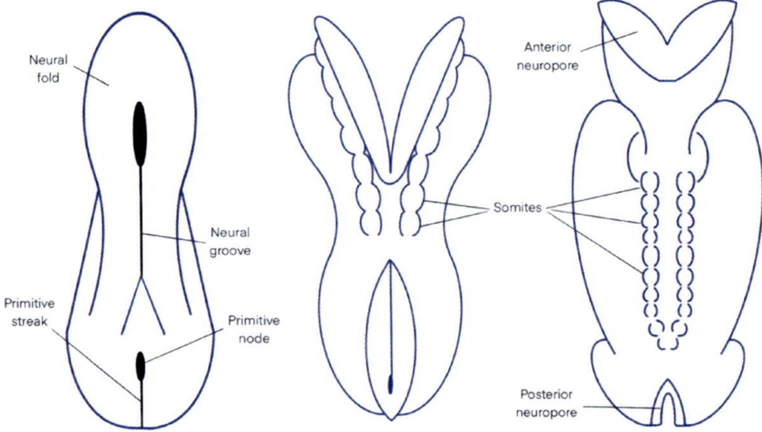

Image 2.16: These particularly unsightly drawings show the process of neurulation from a dorsal view (looking at the "pancake" from the top).

2.8 The folding of the three layer "pancake" into a body

It's as simple as the heading. The three-layer germ disc folds into itself to form two internal tubes (neural tube and primitive gut). It keeps folding until its outer surface is ectoderm (skin). The "pancake" is now an actual body!

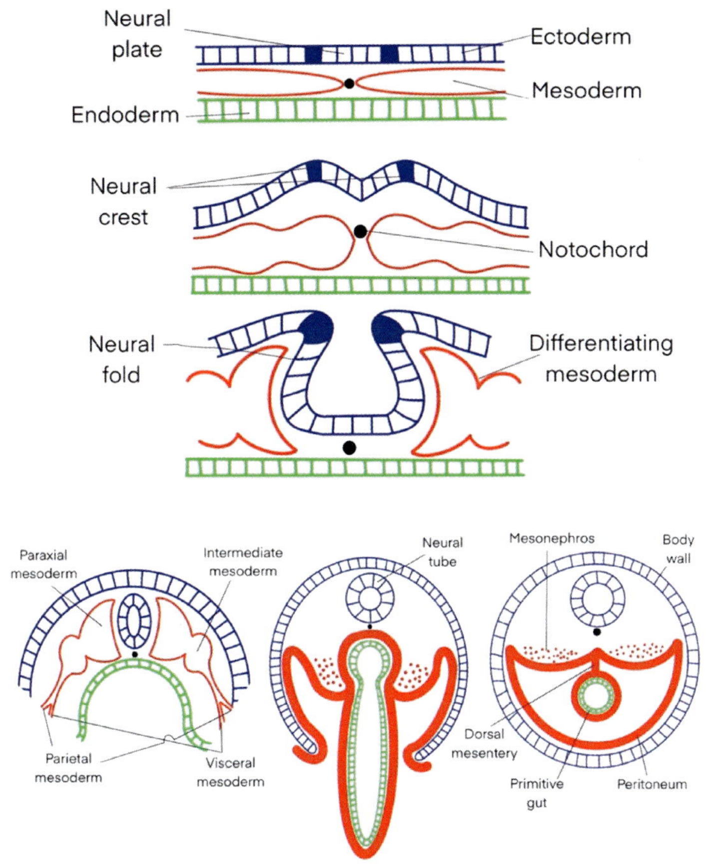

Image 2.17: It's amazing how much growth occurs in 10 days. These cross-sections of the embryo summarise the action between day 18 (top) and day 28 (bottom-right).

2.9 Where everything comes from

Now that we know how the three germ layers are produced from the epiblast by gastrulation, and how the trilaminar disc then folds into a body, it is time to find out what each layer contributes in terms of organ development. This is summarised in Image 2.18.

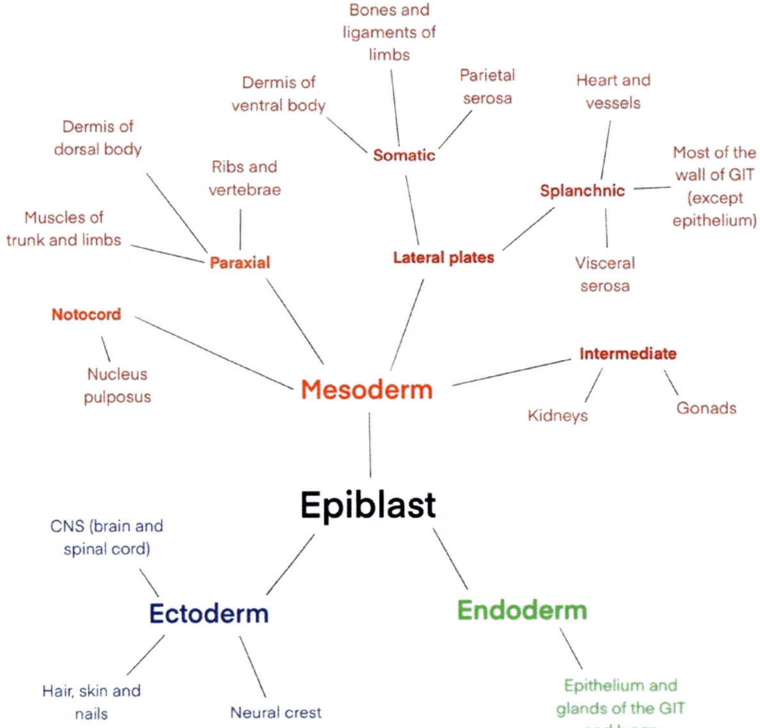

Image 2.18: The tree of foetal life!

Chapter 3: The Heart and Blood Vessels

Initially the embryo gets nutrients via diffusion, but sometime during the third week, diffusion is no longer enough for the growing embryo. Thus, a vascular system begins to develop for the embryo to continue its growth. This chapter will describe the development of said vascular system.

3.1 The Heart

Similar to how cells came in through the primitive streak to create the three germ layers during gastrulation, progenitor heart cells originating at the epiblast enter through the streak and they make their way to the splanchnic lateral plate mesoderm. It is at this location that these cells form the primary heart field. The primary heart field develops into the left ventricle, both atria, and contributes partially to the right ventricle.

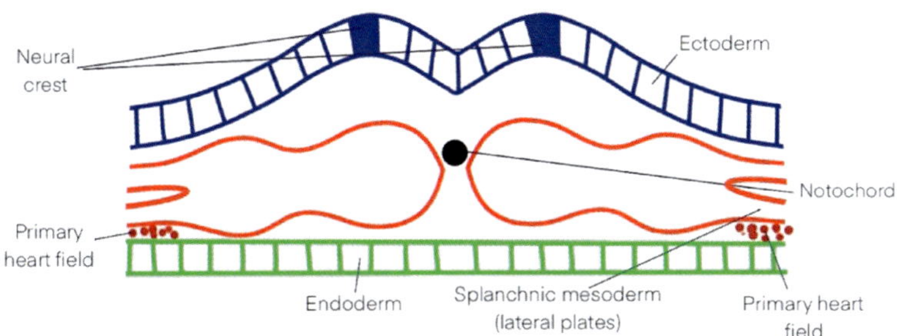

Image 3.1: Cross-section of the embryo illustrating the location of the primary heart field.

The secondary heart field appears by the end of the third week and contributes to the rest of the heart. It is responsible for lengthening the outflow tract of the heart one cell at a time. That is, it lengthens the heart from above like sand filling an hourglass (Image 3.2).

High Yield!

Quick points on the development of the heart:

- The atrioventricular junction becomes the atrioventricular canal
- The bulbis cordis becomes the trabeculated portion of the right ventricle
- The conus cordis becomes the ventricular outflow tracts and
- Truncus arteriosus becomes the aortic root, the ascending aorta, and the pulmonary artery.

Cardiac myoblasts and blood islands are formed by the primary heart field. Eventually the blood islands will join to make a tube that is covered in myoblasts (called the cardiogenic region). Blood islands not only develop within the cardiogenic region, but also on either side of it. These blood islands will also form a pair of tubes called the dorsal aortae.

As the embryo folds laterally (with the sides coming in like a hug) and cephalocaudally (folding in the direction of head-to-toe) the two dorsal aortae fuse with each other except at their lowest zones, and the cardiogenic region grows. At this point, the heart is a big tube with an inner layer of endothelium and an outer layer of muscle (myocardium). There is a third outer layer that is called the epicardium which is developed from the hearts outflow tract. The coronary arteries pop-out from the epicardium. Venous blood comes in from the bottom of the heart and the blood is pumped out from the top to the dorsal aorta. Meanwhile, a process of cardiac looping occurs, where the cardiac tube bends as shown in Images 3.3 and 3.4.

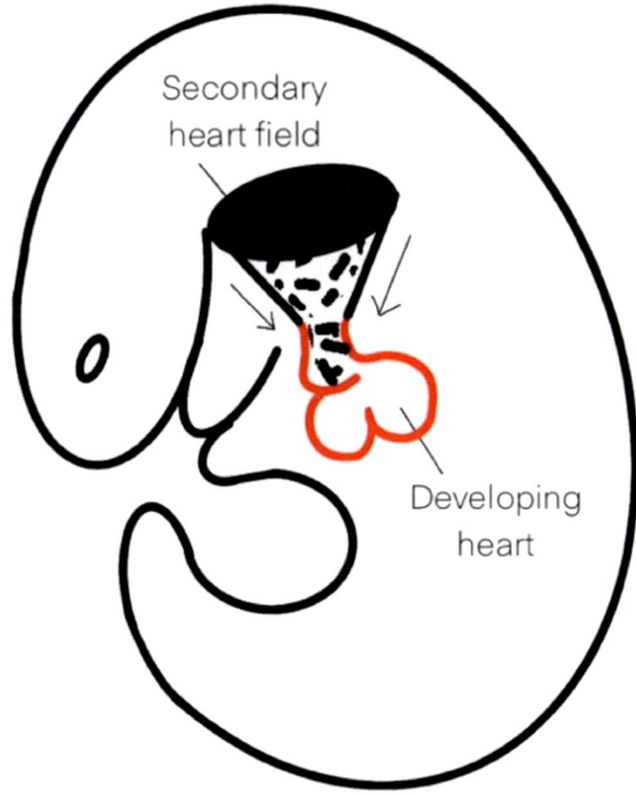

Image 3.2: The heart is lengthened like sand filling an hourglass.

The left and right atria are initially one single cavity, but the human heart has two atriums. So how does the atrium get divided into two cavities? It all starts when a growth of tissue from the roof of the heart called the septum primum (translation: the first septum) grows downwards. The ostium primum (translation: the first door) is the space between the septum primum and the floor of the atrium.

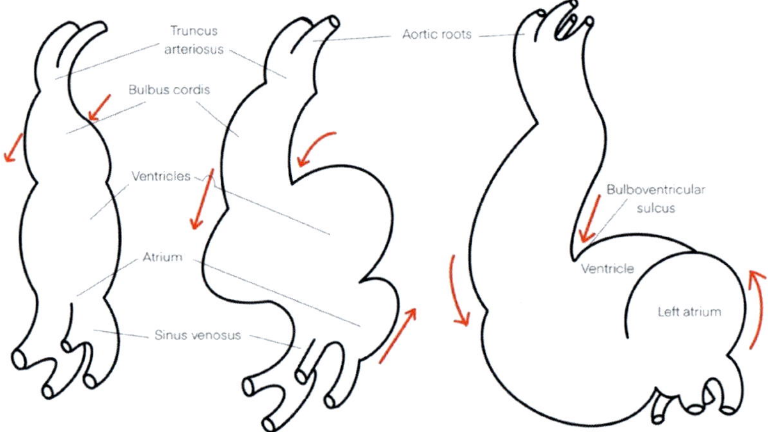

Image 3.3: Cardiac looping: the top of the tube bends down towards the front and to the right. The bottom part of the tube does the opposite, it bends up towards the back and to the left.

Before full fusion, cell death occurs in the septum primum near the roof which forms the ostium secondum to keep blood flowing from the right to the left. Next, a septum secondum forms near the original growth site of the septum primum (in the right atrium) and grows down leaving an opening when it reaches the ostium secondum. This is called the foramen ovale (translation: the oval foramen or the oval hole). Prior to birth, the foramen ovale acts as a valve that allows blood to flow from the right to the left atrium. However, at birth when breathing begins, there is a pressure increase in the left atrium which pushes the valve against the septum secondum causing it to fuse so that blood is no longer shunted from right to left.

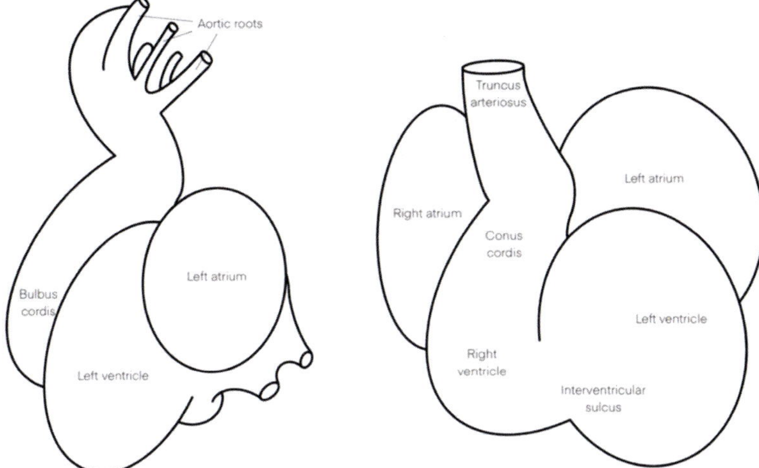

Image 3.4: This is what the heart looks like on day 28 of development. The image on the left is a lateral view of the heart (looking at it sideways from the left side), and the right side is a frontal view. The bulbus cordis (left) is made up of the truncus arteriosus, conus cordis, and part of the right ventricle (right).

High Yield!

By the end of the fourth week of development, the septa of the heart begins development in either of the following ways:

1. There are two separate and opposite facing growing pieces of tissue, called the endocardial cushions, that meet and fuse together. The atrial and ventricular septa are divided like this.
2. Two growing walls of the heart move towards each other, and then their cells proliferate causing them to fuse. The atria and ventricles are divided like this.

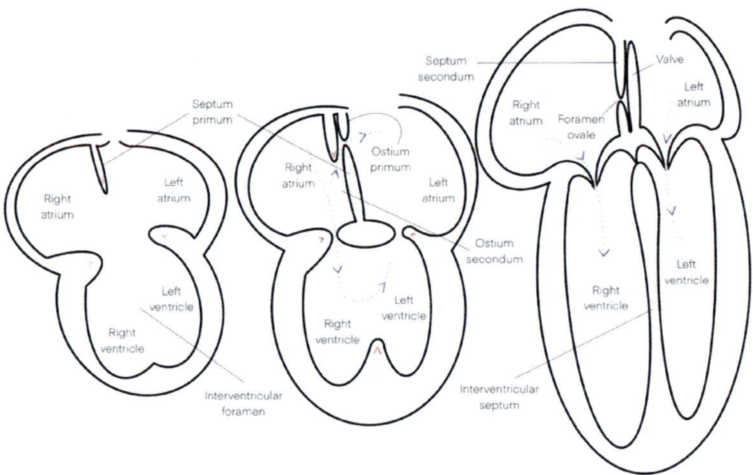

Image 3.5: Development of the atrial and ventricular septa.

High Yield!

The pulmonary vein comes from the back of the left atrial wall and joins with veins that are growing from the developing lungs. These veins become part of the left atrium, and this process forms the smooth walled part of the atrium.

At the end of the first month, growths of tissue called the atrioventricular endocardial cushions grow from the front and the back of the atrioventricular canal. In addition, there are two lateral atrioventricular endocardial cushions growing into the lumen which fuse together like shown in Image 3.5.

After fusion of the endocardial cushions, the flow of blood disintegrates some tissue lining the ventricles to form the valves. Think of rain over thousands of years and how it erodes and shapes rocks and cliffs. This is a similar process to how blood hollows out the ventricles to form the valves. The valves are connected to the ventricle wall by papillary muscles via cordae tendinae. This is how the mitral and tricuspid valves form.

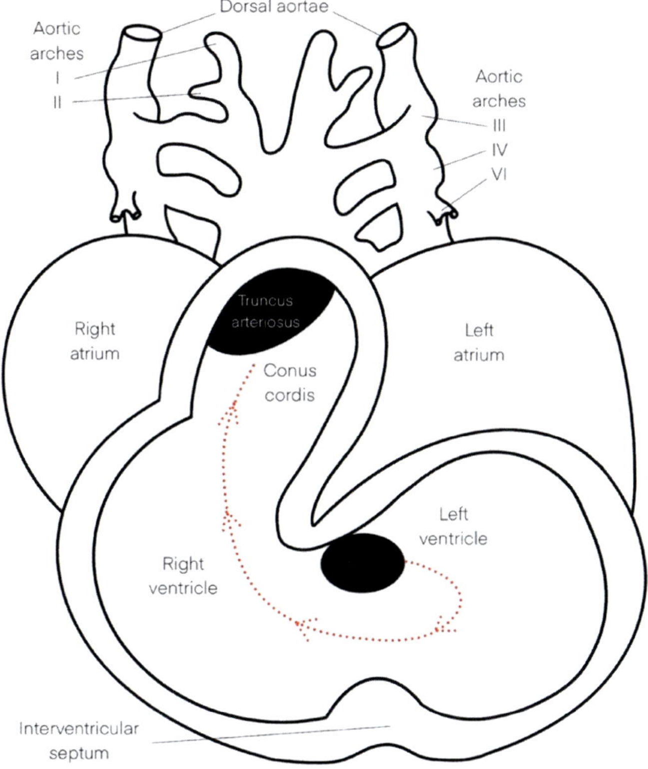

Image 3.6: Day 30: a frontal section of heart. Blood flows from the atrioventricular canal to the truncus arteriosus in the direction shown by the red arrow. The aortic arches are the arteries of the pharyngeal arches.

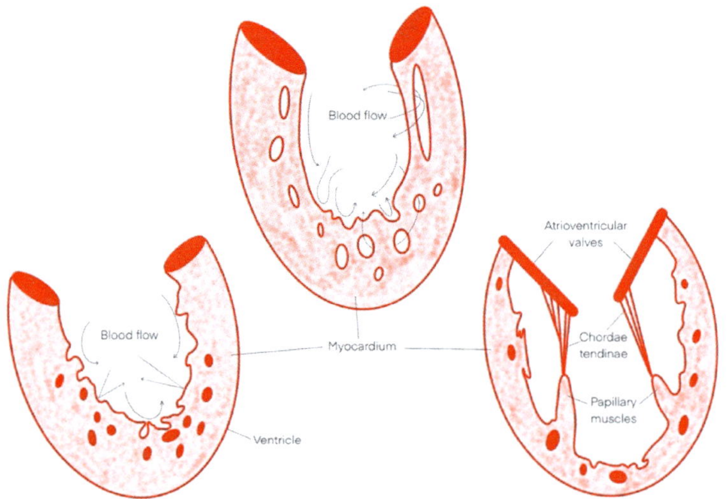

Image 3.7: Cross-section of a ventricle. Blood flow through the ventricles (indicated by black arrows) destroy some of the myocardium until all that remains are the valves, chordae tendineae, and the papillary muscle. Brutal, yet necessary.

Arterial and venous blood flow are separated when a septum forms in the truncus arteriosus and conus cordis. Inside the truncus during the second month, more tissue cushions grow from the right upper wall and on the left lower wall. The right cushion grows down and left and the left cushion does the opposite while twisting around each other and completely fusing. This is now called the aorticopulmonary septum and the truncus is split into an aortic and pulmonary tube.

A similar process occurs in the conus cordis, where cushions grow and fuse together and with the aorticopulmonary septum. At this point, the conus is split into the outflow tract of the right ventricle and the outflow tract of the left ventricle.

As the ventricles expand, the interventricular septum is formed by the merging of the walls of the ventricles.

3.2 Arteries

Formation of the arteries are related to the pharyngeal arches (see Chapter 9 for the pharyngeal arches). Each arch is gifted a nerve and an artery. The arteries are called aortic arches and they come from the truncus arteriosus.

These arches first appear from the top, that is, arch I appears first, then arch II, and so on. The fifth arch does not contribute to anything, so there are five arches, but they are labelled to VI skipping V which disappears into oblivion.

The first aortic arch becomes the maxillary artery, and the second aortic arch becomes the hyoid and stapedial arteries. The third aortic arch forms the common carotid artery, the external carotid artery, and a portion of the internal carotid artery. The fourth aortic arch on the left becomes the aortic arch, and on the right forms a portion of the right subclavian artery. Finally, the sixth aortic arch is the pulmonary arch. They become the pulmonary arteries, but the left one has the honour of also forming the ductus arteriosus. The rest of the internal carotid artery comes from the dorsal aorta.

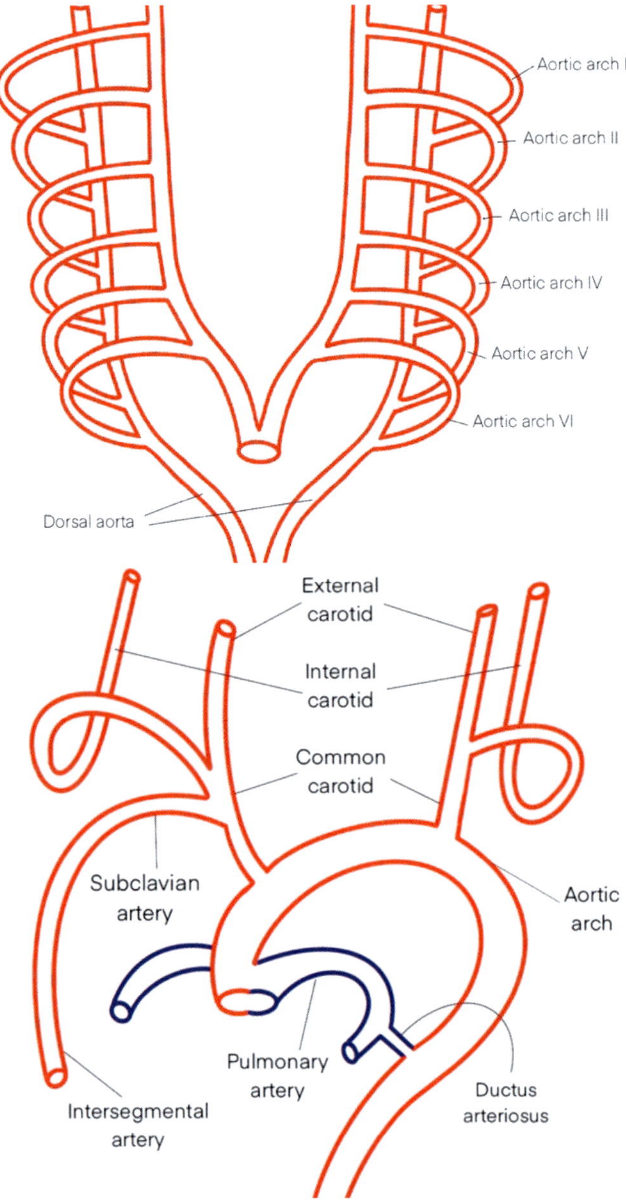

Image 3.8: Two snapshots in time during the development of the aortic arches. Top: the arches prior to any differentiation. Bottom: Notice how the ductus arteriosus is patent at this time.

3.3 The Coronary Arteries

The coronary arteries are created from the epicardium as well as from angioblasts that grow off the sinus venosus. These vessels grow into the aorta behind the aortic valve (the left and right coronary cusps). Blood flows into the coronary arteries during diastole because the coronary cusps close off the opening to the coronary vessels during systole and accept the backflow of blood during diastole (like an upside-down umbrella in a storm).

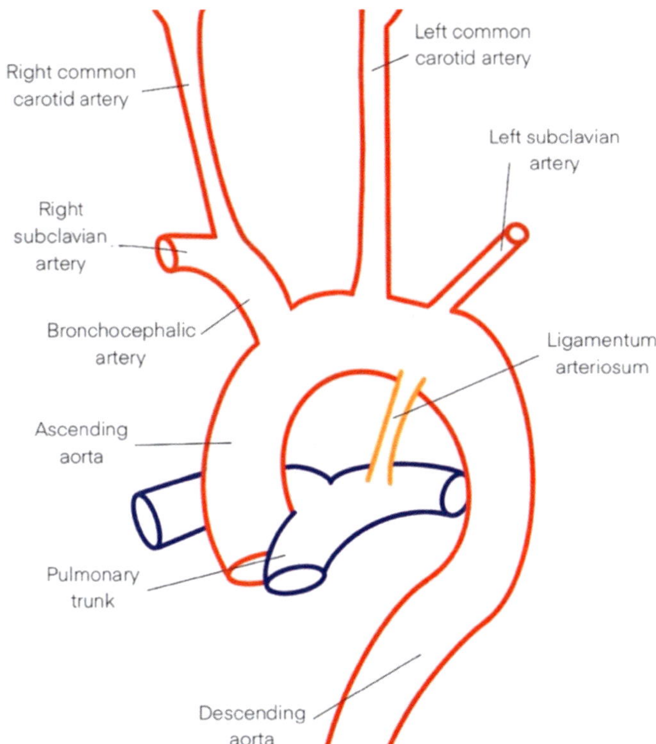

Image 3.9: The final form of the great arteries.

3.4 Veins

Vitelline and allantois are two new words to learn in this subchapter. To keep it simple, just learn the word and associate it to the structure (look at Image 3.10). The vitelline veins bring blood from the yolk sac to the sinus venosus. Although some of it disappears into another dimension, the parts that remain forms some of the inferior vena cava, the portal vein, and superior mesenteric vein. The vitelline vein plexus that surrounds the duodenum enters the septum transversum and then the sinus venosus. Eventually the plexus surrounding the duodenum becomes the portal vein, and the right vitelline vein develops into the superior mesenteric vein.

The umbilical veins bring oxygenated blood to the developing embryo from the placenta. Like the vitelline veins, some of the umbilical veins also disappear. Only the left umbilical vein remains which communicates to the rest of the system via the ductus venosus. The ductus venosus shunts blood away from the liver. After birth the umbilical vein and ductus venosus become ligaments (ligamentum teres and venosum respectively).

The cardinal veins are the draining veins. It initially consists of a common, an anterior, and a posterior cardinal vein. The anterior vein drains the top part of the embryo, and the posterior drains the bottom.

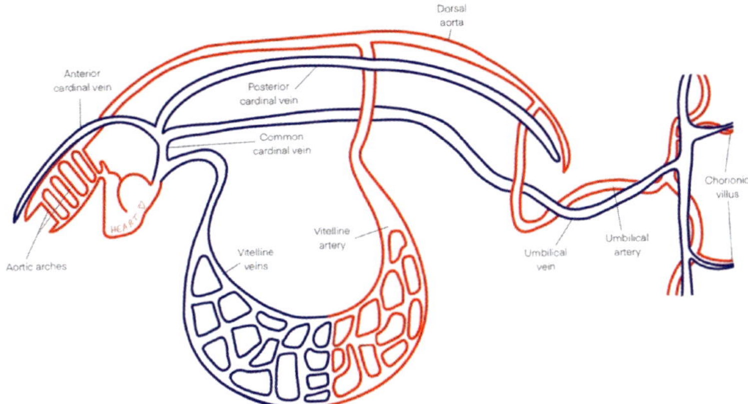

Image 3.10: The circulatory system of a foetus in the fifth week.

Chapter 4: The Respiratory System

Chapter 4 is relatively short because we discuss the development of the lungs in a simple manner. Let's get straight into it.

4.1 The Lungs

During the fourth week, the lung bud turns up as a protrusion from the gastrointestinal tract. This growth is triggered by retinoic acid released by mesodermal cells.

As the lung bud grows down, the tracheoesophageal ridges form, closing the lung bud off from the gut/oesophagus. The tracheoesophageal ridges are the grooves that appear when one tube is pinching off another one to form two tubes.

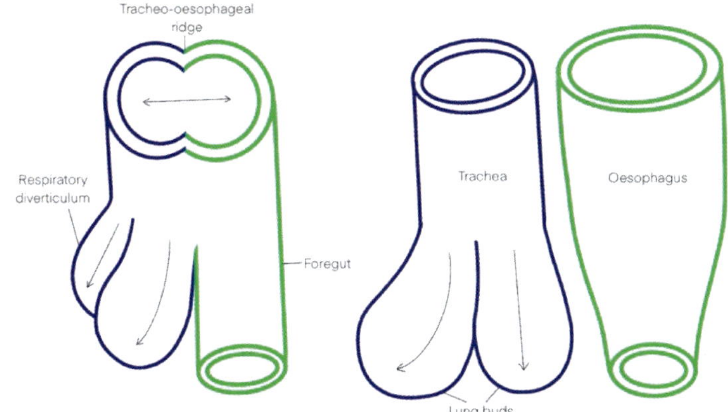

Image 4.1: The respiratory diverticulum "pinching off" the foregut to become the trachea with its lung buds, and the oesophagus.

Cartilage and muscle of the larynx comes from the fourth and sixth pharyngeal arches. The fifth pharyngeal arch does not contribute to much as we will learn in Chapter 9. The vocal cords are formed when two growths from the larynx, aptly called the laryngeal growths, appear following canalisation of the larynx.

The lung bud becomes the trachea and bronchioles. Just as the lung buds grow off the foregut, the bronchial buds grow off the lung buds. The bronchial buds become the left and right main bronchi by week five. Eventually the right bronchus will divide into three secondary bronchi corresponding to the three lobes of the right lung, and the left bronchus into two secondary bronchi. These lung buds continue to grow until all the space in the chest is taken up. The pleura comes from the lateral plate mesoderm (visceral pleura from splanchnic and parietal from somatic).

High Yield!

Inhalation actually begins before birth and the foetus inhales some of the amniotic fluid. This allows for development of the breathing muscles. At birth, most of the fluid is absorbed leaving behind only the surfactant in a healthy baby.

The three secondary bronchi on the right become ten tertiary bronchi and the two on the left become eight, and these subsequently continue branching out until the terminal bronchus form the respiratory bronchioles. A bonus division by the respiratory bronchioles forms alveolar ducts. These ducts are covered in alveolar cells, of which there are two types. Type 1 alveolar cells are flat cells surrounded by blood vessels and are responsible for the exchange of gases.

Type 2 alveolar cells are the surfactant producing cells. Surfactant is important in allowing the pleura to freely glide over each other without tension.

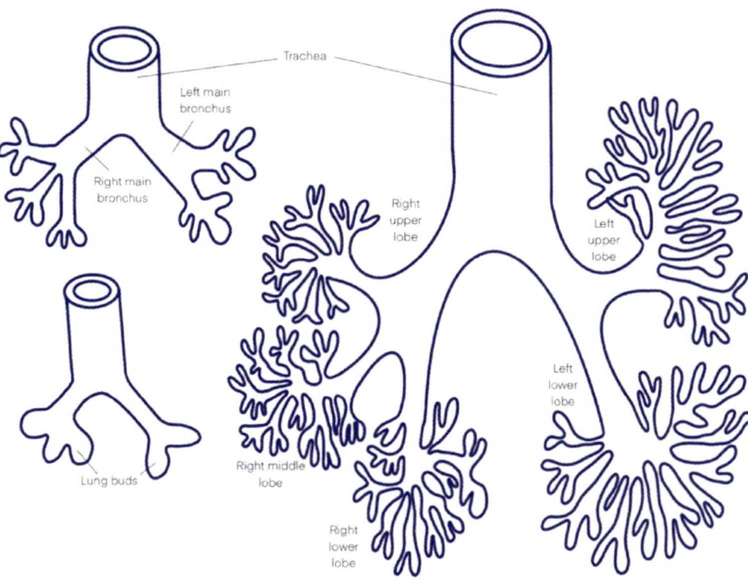

Image 4.2: The lung buds grow to fill the chest cavity and form the lobes of the lung by branching into smaller and smaller bronchioles. There is no "left middle lobe" rather, the equivalent area in the left lung is called the lingula. The left lung has 2 lobes, the upper and lower.

Chapter 5: The Gastrointestinal System

The gut tube is formed by endoderm (epithelium and glands), and splanchnic mesoderm (connective tissue and musculature).

This chapter will be broken down into the following three parts, top-to-bottom, literally:

1. The foregut (we also discuss the surrounding organs)
2. The midgut and
3. The hindgut.

5.1 The Foregut

The foregut consists of the oesophagus, stomach and duodenum. It extends from the mouth to the major papilla of the duodenum. Its blood supply is from the coeliac trunk.

5.1.1 Oesophagus

The oesophagus and the lungs both develop from the lung bud, which appears during week four. Growth of tissue separates the trachea from the oesophagus. As the lungs and heart grow and move deeper into the thoracic cavity, the oesophagus is also pulled down and becomes longer. The epithelium of the oesophagus is endoderm, and the muscles come from splanchnic mesoderm. The upper portion of the oesophagus is striated muscle, and the lower portion is smooth muscle.

5.1.2 Stomach

The stomach develops as a foregut dilatation during week four. The stomach undergoes changes in its position, size, and shape, and it rotates along two axes. One is the longitudinal axis (turning around a vertical line) and the other is the anteroposterior axis (like leaning back or picking something off the ground).

Along the longitudinal axis, the stomach rotates 90 degrees clockwise while at the same time the posterior portion of the stomach grows faster than the anterior portion. This process forms the greater and lesser curvatures. Now imagine, since the posterior portion is much larger than the anterior, that the stomach is forced to lean back into its final position. This "leaning back" is the rotation along the anteroposterior axis that the stomach makes to find its final position.

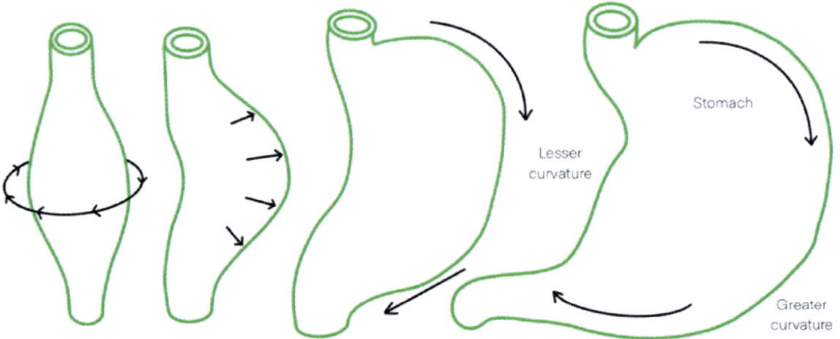

Image 5.1: The development of the stomach.

The stomach is attached to the back of the body by the dorsal mesogastrium and to the front by the ventral mesogastrium. During the rotation described above, the stomach pulls both the dorsal and ventral mesogastrium resulting in the dorsal mesogastrium being pushed down and to the left. As it is being pushed down, the dorsal mesogastrium also grows into a covering that extends over most of the colon and the small intestines. It remains connected to the greater curvature of the stomach. This is the greater omentum. The ventral mesogastrium develops into both the lesser omentum and the falciform ligament.

5.1.3 Duodenum

The junction between the foregut and the midgut, at the major duodenal papilla, is the location of where the liver buds form. Duodenal rotation is influenced by stomach rotation such that as the stomach rotates, the duodenum loops into its characteristic shape. This rotation puts the duodenum in a retroperitoneal location.

Cells in the duodenum undergo proliferation halfway through the first trimester that clog the entire tube up. This is the solid stage of duodenal development. However, the solid stage of development is short-lived, as the cells end up disintegrating to recreate a patent lumen.

5.1.4 Liver

During the third week, the liver bud, which is also known as the hepatic diverticulum, begins to grow from the endoderm at the junction of the foregut and midgut. The liver bud penetrates the septum transversum (mesoderm) and the bile duct is formed because of the thinning of the connection between the liver bud and the duodenum. The gallbladder and cystic duct grow from the bile duct, and the hepatic sinusoids appear when liver cells form connections with the umbilical and vitelline veins. Stem cells, Kupffer cells and stromal cells are all developed from the septum transversum. The septum will go on to become the central tendon of the diaphragm.

High Yield!

The peritoneal covering of the liver comes from mesoderm. The liver is covered by peritoneum except where it comes into contact with the diaphragm (the bare area).

5.1.5 Pancreas

In contrast to the single liver bud that becomes the liver, the pancreas begins as two buds. These are the ventral and dorsal pancreatic buds, and in the beginning, these are on opposite sides of the foregut. As the stomach and duodenum rotates clockwise, the ventral bud moves towards the dorsal bud coming to its final position below and behind the dorsal pancreatic bud. The ducts and pancreatic tissue of the ventral and dorsal bud fuse and the uncinate process of the pancreas is formed. The duct of Wirsung, the main pancreatic duct, is developed from the ventral bud and the distal dorsal bud. The duct of Santorini, the accessory duct, is from the proximal dorsal pancreatic bud. Thus, the duct of Wirsung has on opening to the duodenum at the major duodenal papilla, and the duct of Santorini has an opening to the duodenum via the minor duodenal papilla.

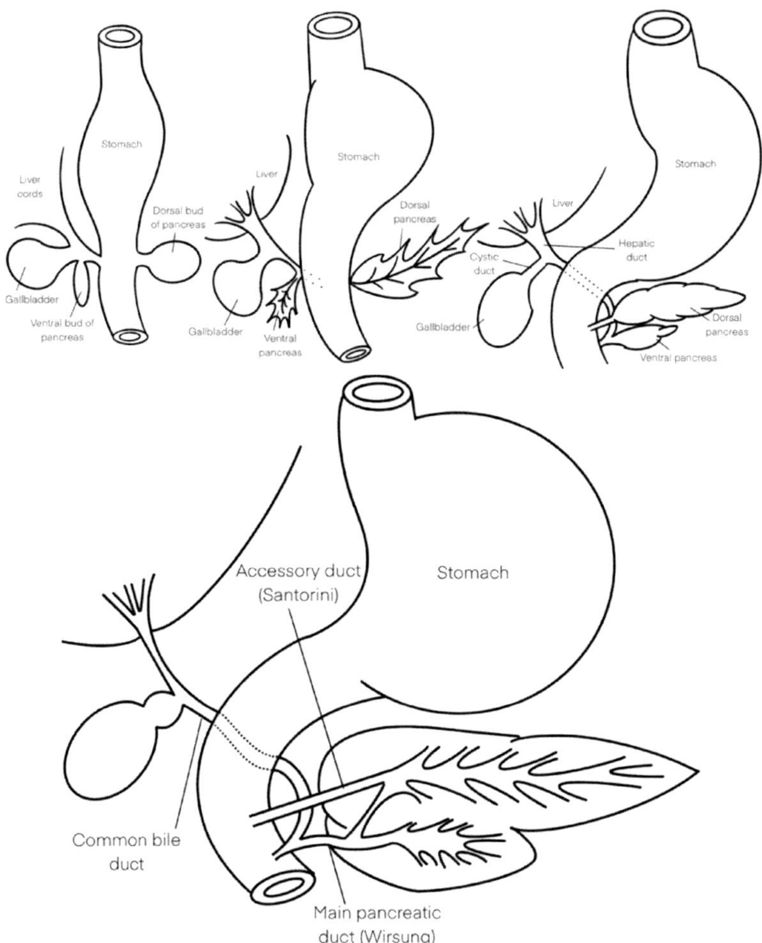

Image 5.2: The development of the pancreas.

5.1.6 Spleen

The spleen begins as a growth from the mesoderm of the dorsal mesogastrium. To picture this, imagine a connection from the rear body wall to the spleen made by the dorsal mesogastrium. Then picture a connection to the stomach from the spleen from the anterior portion of the dorsal mesogastrium. As the stomach keeps rotating and the spleen grows the dorsal mesogastrium continues to stretch, putting the spleen in its final position to the left of the abdomen. Mesodermal cells contribute to form the cells of the spleen, including the capsule and connective tissue.

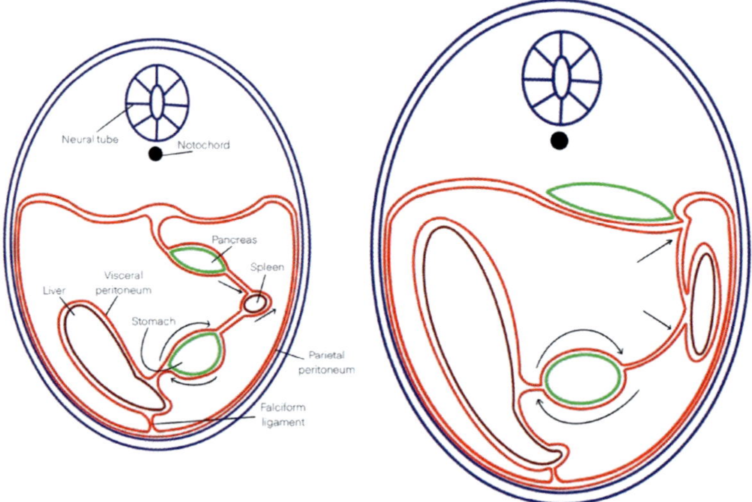

Image 5.3: Cross-section of the growing foetus at the level of the rotating stomach, spleen, pancreas, and liver. Arrows show the movement of the connective tissue that joins all the organs in the abdominal wall.

5.2 The Midgut

The midgut is a long tube that extends from the major papilla of the duodenum to the junction of the proximal two-thirds of the transverse colon with the distal third. Its blood supply is from the superior mesenteric artery and initially it is in open communication with the yolk sac via the vitelline duct.

The midgut becomes longer very quickly during its development. However, it wasn't always known as a midgut. Initially the midgut was known as the primary intestinal loop. The primary intestinal loop has two parts to it and is defined by its location relative to the connection with the vitelline duct (see Image 5.4 to visualise this). There is a cephalic (superior) limb, and a caudal (inferior) limb. The cephalic limb becomes the duodenum, jejunum, and the proximal ileum. The caudal limb becomes the rest of the ileum, caecum including appendix, and up to the first two-thirds of the transverse colon.

The primary intestinal loop rotates around the superior mesenteric artery, for a total of 270 degrees counterclockwise. During the rotation the small intestine continues to grow longer and become coiled, and the large intestine becomes longer without coiling. As the primary intestinal loop rotates and elongates, it is pushed out of the abdominal cavity (physiological herniation) by the growing liver. For perspective, 90 degrees of the rotation occurs during physiological herniation, and the remaining rotation occurs as the midgut returns to the abdomen. Physiological herniation essentially refers to a type of herniation that is not pathological, a "normal" herniation, hence physiological herniation.

The order in which the herniated loops of intestines make their way back into the abdomen explains their final position in the abdomen. For example, the jejunum is the first back into the abdomen, thus it lies on the left side. The caecum initially lies in the right upper quadrant of the abdomen since it is the last to re-enter. Following re-entry, the caecum descends pulling the ascending colon with it. The appendix is formed when a portion of the distal caecum proliferates into a tube during the migration of the caecum.

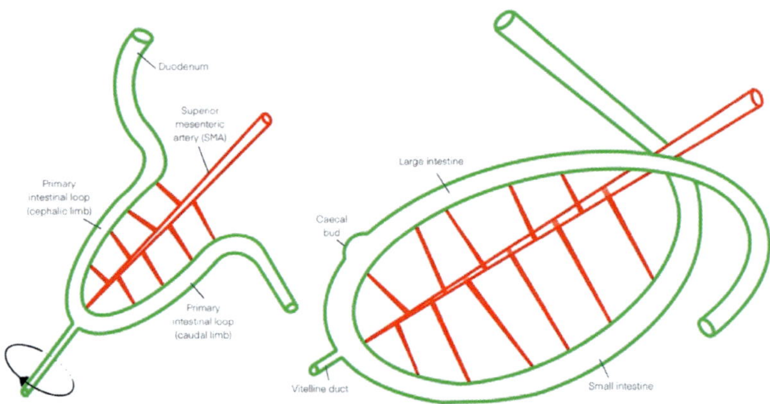

Image 5.4: Rotation of the midgut along its axis, the superior mesenteric artery.

5.3 The Hindgut

The hindgut develops into the distal third of the transverse colon, the descending colon, the sigmoid colon, and the rectum. In addition to its gastrointestinal contribution, the hindgut endoderm contributes to the epithelium of the bladder and urethra. The hindgut is supplied by the inferior mesenteric artery.

Introducing a new word for your vocabulary: the cloaca. The cloaca is a cavity that is lined with endoderm on the inside, and ectoderm on the front surface. Divide the cloaca into two parts, an anterior portion which is in open communication with the allantois, and a posterior portion which is in open communication with the hindgut. The junction between the endoderm and ectoderm parts is called the cloacal membrane.

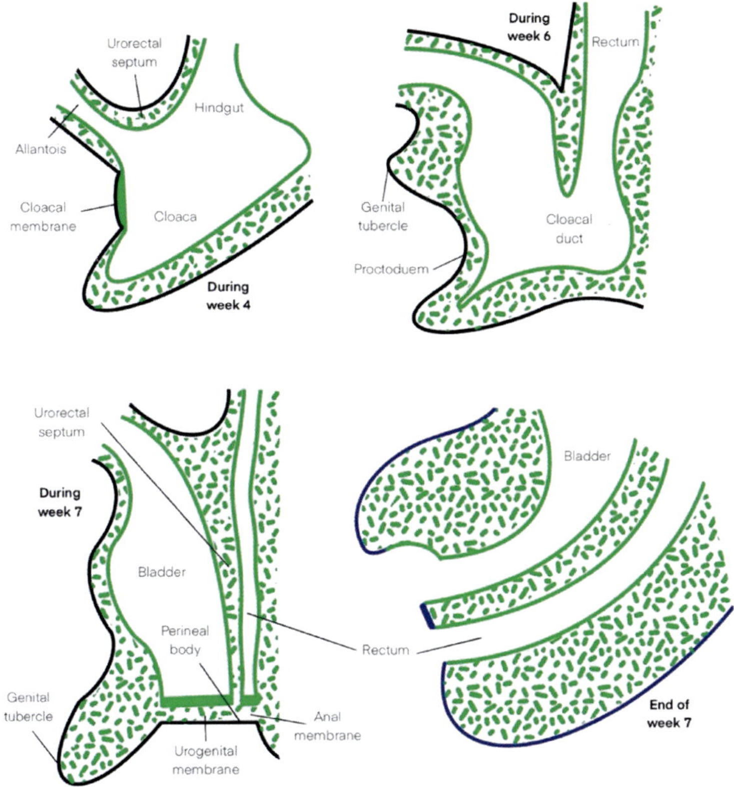

Image 5.5: The development of the hindgut. Keep this image in mind when reviewing the urinary system in Chapter 6.

The urorectal septum, which is mesoderm, separates the allantois and the hindgut. The continued folding of the embryo pushes the urorectal septum down towards the cloacal membrane and by week eight the membrane opens to form an anal opening and an opening for the urinary tract. The end of the urogenital septum becomes the perineal body which separates the anal opening from the genital opening.

Both ectoderm and endoderm contribute to the rectum. The inferior third of the rectum is derived from ectoderm that penetrates inside the body, whereas the upper two-thirds is derived from the endoderm of the hindgut. The boundary separating these is called the pectinate line. An important line to know of if you'd like to be a colorectal surgeon, or if you are a colorectal surgeon and you want to quiz your medical students while performing the gruesome task of a haemorrhoidectomy (true story).

Chapter 6: The Renal System and Adrenals

Chapter 6 is divided into three parts:

1. First, we talk about the kidneys
2. Then we go over adrenals briefly because of the proximity rule
3. Finally, we discuss the bladder, urethra, and prostate.

Even though the gonads are derived from the same part of the mesoderm as the renal system, we discuss the sex organs in the next chapter.

6.1 The Kidneys

The kidney doesn't evolve from the same ball of cells like some of the other organs or a Pokémon. However, like most Pokémon, the kidneys have three stages of development. The pronephros is the first stage and is a rudimentary structure. This means that it is not a functioning kidney, nor does it develop into anything, rather it disappears into another universe. The second stage, the mesonephros, only functions as a filtration system for a limited time. Its arguable that everything in life is for a limited time, but there is a third stage of kidney development that takes over from the mesonephros. The third stage is the metanephros and it is this structure that forms the final form of the kidney. The Charizard of the kidney.

Kidney development in the form of a pronephros begins in week four, but all that has developed in this stage completely disappears by the end of this week. Image 6.1 is not a single snapshot in time, rather it makes up all three stages in one image, so it might be easier to understand if you imagine a blind is being pulled down slowly over the image from the top, and at this rate the top of the image is degenerated, making way for the more mature versions of the kidney at the bottom. The top of the pronephros begins to degenerate and in one week it is completely gone, but as this happens the metanephros takes over, and so on.

The mesonephros is the stage where mesonephric ducts and tubules develop. These develop while the pronephros degenerates. That is, as the blind comes down putting the pronephros to sleep, the mesonephros develops. The mesonephric tubules are the first excretory tubules that grow. They grow quickly and take a squiggly line shape like a tilde (tilde is the ~ character). Blood supply via capillaries forms the glomerulus and Bowman's capsule is formed by the mesonephric tubules. This is the renal corpuscle. These tubules drain into the mesonephric duct, which is also known as the Wolffian duct. The development of the mesonephros is from the top to the bottom. So as the lower mesonephric tubules develop the ones on the top start to degenerate, and at the end of week eight the mesonephric tubules disappear completely in the female, but in the male some of the mesonephros is involved in gonad formation (see Chapter 7).

The metanephros is the final form of the kidney. The metanephros is what is left in your body right now as you're reading this line. It begins to form in week five when the ureteric bud begins to grow from the mesonephric duct. As dilatation of the bud occurs, the renal pelvis is beginning to take shape and begins its division into the major calyces. The major calyces form tubules as they grow further into the tissue like tree roots. This continues until week 20. The minor calyces are formed by the continued enlargement of the tubules near the major calyces.

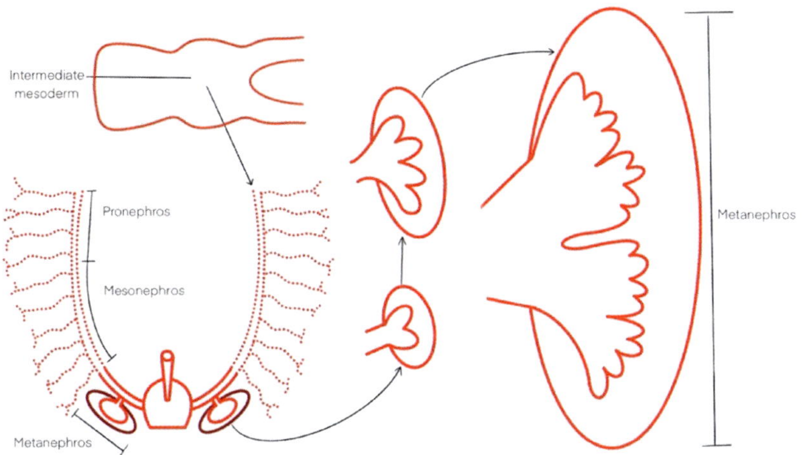

Image 6.1: It is incredibly difficult to simplify the embryology of the kidney into a picture, but this image is the best attempt. The image on the bottom-left describes the entire process. Keep in mind that this picture is not a single snapshot in time, rather the combination of all three stages of kidney development over many weeks. The dotted line means the structures do not contribute to the final form of the kidney.

The tubules have an end covered with tissue that is called the metanephric tissue cap. The metanephric tissue cap forms the renal vesicles that become tubules and capillaries (the glomeruli). This is now known as the nephron. Bowman's capsule is formed by the tip of the nephron, and the other end of the nephron forms a connection with the collecting tubules. The nephron continues to lengthen to form the proximal convoluted tubule, the loop of Henle, and the distal convoluted tubule. The development of the nephron continues after birth. No more nephrons are created, but the existing nephrons continue to become larger for a few more years.

High Yield!

The final form of the kidney is, at first, a pelvic organ. However, as the body grows continuously, the kidneys move into their final position inside the abdomen.

6.2 The Adrenal Glands

The adrenal glands are derived from mesoderm and ectoderm. The mesoderm contributes to the cortex of the adrenal glands, and the ectoderm to the medulla. Neuroblasts (see Chapter 8) that are involved in the development of the sympathetic nervous system will form the primitive cortex. Another wave of cells then arrives and surrounds the primitive cortex forming the adrenal glands definitive cortex. The primitive cortex will become the zona reticularis. The neural crest cells contribute to the medulla of the adrenals (the chromaffin cells).

6.3 Bladder, Urethra, and Prostate

The cloaca divides into the urogenital sinus and anal canal. These are divided by the descending urorectal septum, which is mesodermal tissue, the tip of which forms the peroneal body (see Image 5.5). The urogenital sinus becomes the bladder, and in males becomes the prostatic urethra (which crosses the prostate) and the membranous urethra (which passes through the external urethral sphincter).

The epithelial cells of the urethra are developed from endoderm, and the smooth muscle cells are derived from the mesoderm. The prostate develops from the prostatic urethra as it proliferates and invades surrounding tissue. In females, this similar part of the urethra becomes the urethral and paraurethral glands. The Gräfenberg spot will be discussed in Easy Embryology: Part 2.

Chapter 7: The Reproductive System

This chapter will be beginning with a brief discussion on sex determination. This is then followed by outlining the "indifferent stage" of development. The indifferent stage is the stage prior to commencement of sexual differentiation into a male, female, or other variants. Then, we will describe the embryology of the reproductive systems, both internally and externally, for both genders.

7.1 Sex

Sex is determined by the Y chromosome which contains the sex-determining region on Y gene (SRY). SRY produces a protein, the SRY protein, which in its absence female development occurs, and in its presence male development occurs.

High Yield!

Sex is determined at fertilisation, but it is at week seven that differentiation into either male or female occurs.

7.2 The Indifferent Stage

7.2.1 Gonads

The gonads are derived from the intermediate mesoderm. They first appear as the gonadal ridges when the underlying epithelial tissue rapidly grows. As mentioned in Chapter 1, germ cells reach the gonadal ridge in week six. The gonads do not develop without these germ cells. The gonadal ridges will continue to grow until they become the primitive sex cords.

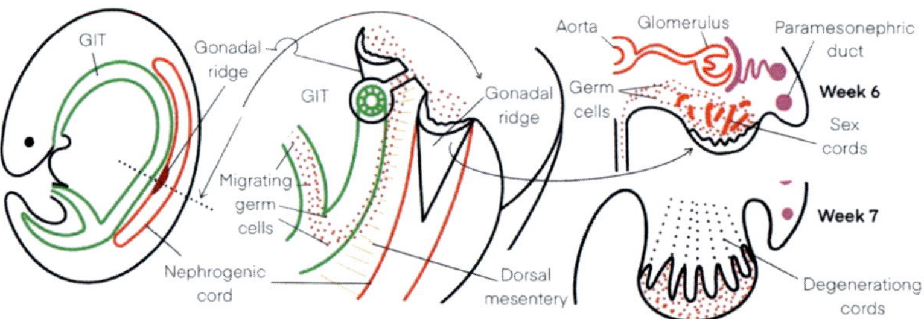

Image 7.1: It's beautiful how the indifferent stage of reproductive embryology can be summarised in one image.

7.2.2 Ducts

At the indifferent stage, the mesonephric ducts and paramesonephric (Mullerian) ducts are present. The mesonephric duct is developed as described in Chapter 6. The paramesonephric duct is created when it pinches off the urogenital ridge, and is the main duct involved in the female reproductive tract development.

7.2.3 The External Organs

The indifferent stage of external genital development begins in week three. Cloacal folds develop when cells enter the cloacal membrane from the primitive streak. At the top end, the genital tubercle is formed when the folds meet. At the bottom there are two folds. One is the urethral and the other is the anal fold. Genital swellings are also formed next to the urethral folds which will become either the scrotum (male) or the labia majora (female). As you can already tell, the external genitals are formed by either some sort of fold or some type of swelling.

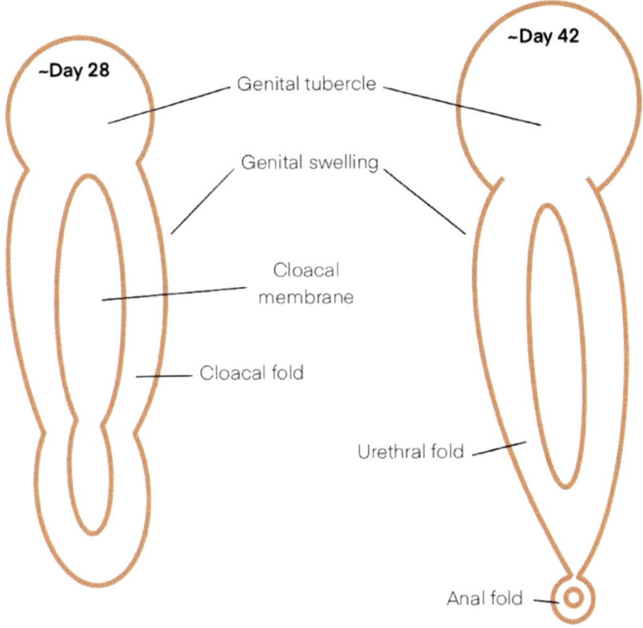

Image 7.2: The indifferent stage of sexual development.

7.3 The Male Reproductive System

7.3.1 The Testis and Ducts

Under the influence of the SRY protein, the primitive sex cords mentioned earlier develop to form the testis (initially as the medullary cords). The sex cords break into tubules called the rete testis. In addition, SRY, SOX9, and steroid genesis factor-1 (SF1) lead to the development of anti-Mullerian hormone which, as the name would suggest, leads to destruction of the Mullerian duct (paramesonephric duct). SRY also triggers the mesonephric tubules to form efferent tubules which join the rete testis and the mesonephric ducts to form the epididymis. The mesonephric ducts then become longer and squiggly, by winding around and overlapping each other. This is how the epididymis is formed. The remainder of the mesonephric tubules form the efferent ducts. As this occurs, the tunica albuginea develops and separates the medullary cords from the epithelium of the testis. These ducts grow muscles and become the ductus deferens. The seminiferous tubules join the efferent duct which connects to the ductus deferens. The ductus deferens develops from the Wolffian duct (mesonephric duct).

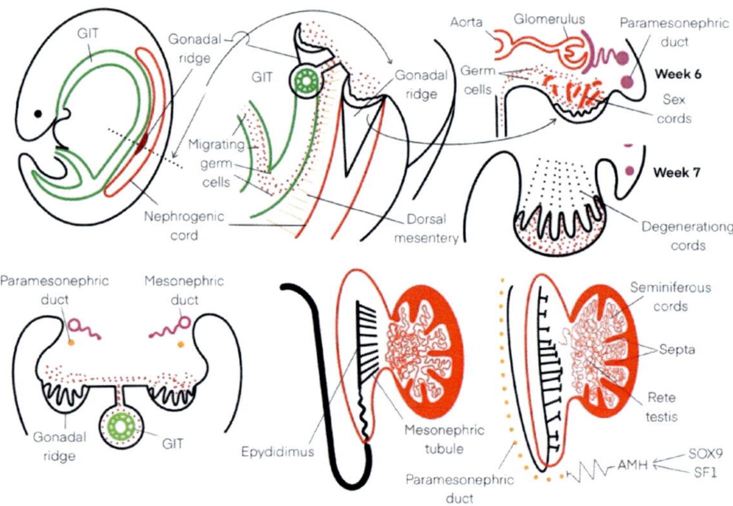

Image 7.3: The development of the testes. The images on the top revisit the indifferent stage. The images on the bottom demonstrate differentiation into testes. Bottom-left is a cross-sectional view. Bottom-centre and bottom-right are sagittal sections.

7.3.2 The Sertoli and Leydig Cells

Sertoli cells develop from the epithelium of the testis and appear during week 20. Leydig cells are developed from the gonadal ridge and at week eight produce testosterone. The function of both cells is described in Chapter 1.

7.3.3 The External Male Reproductive System

The genital swellings are called the scrotal swellings once male differentiation occurs. They grow and descend with each swelling contributing to their half of the scrotum. The genital tubercle quickly becomes longer and is called the phallus, this elongation causes the phallus to pull the urethral folds which now form the edges of the urethral groove. There are individual differences in the degree of elongation of the phallus, with some males getting the short end of the stick. The urethral groove epithelium, which is derived from endoderm, develops into the urethral plate. The folds close over the plates and the urethra is formed by week 12. The tip of the urethra becomes patent between weeks 14-16 when ectoderm from the surface enters at the tip to form the external urethral meatus.

High Yield!

It is at puberty that the seminiferous cords become the seminiferous tubules. That is, the seminiferous cords will finally develop a lumen during puberty.

The lower edge of the testis and the inguinal region between external and internal oblique muscles are connected to the gubernaculum. The gubernaculum is a string of tissue that helps the testis descend into its final position in the scrotum.

The testis passes into the inguinal ring on its descent from the abdomen reaching the scrotum at 33 weeks. Its blood supply is still from the aorta. The processus vaginalis is a part of the peritoneum that follows the gubernaculum into the scrotum. It pulls muscle and connective tissue and voilà the inguinal canal is formed.

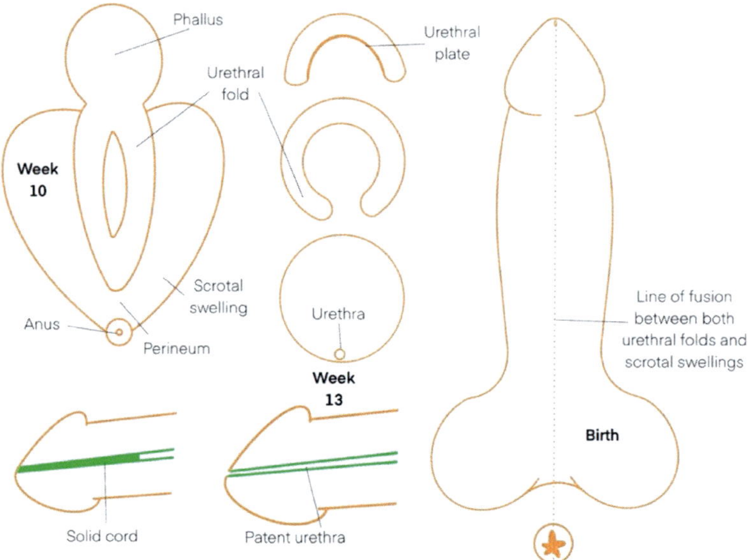

Image 7.4: Development of the penis and scrotum.

7.4 The Female Reproductive System

7.4.1 The Ovary and Ducts

In the absence of a Y chromosome (in the presence of two X chromosomes) female development occurs. The primitive sex cords will become clusters of cells which contain the primitive germ cells. Eventually this becomes the ovarian medulla. The epithelium of the future ovary develops into the cortical cords. In week 12, these cords become cell clusters which continue to grow surrounding the oogonium with follicular cells. This is the primordial follicle. The ovaries do descend, but obviously not to the extent of the testis.

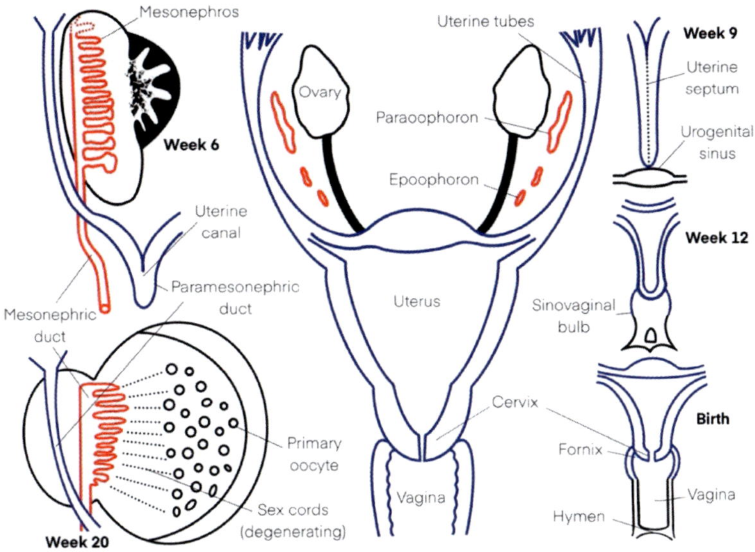

Image 7.5: Development of the ovaries, uterus, and vagina.

The paramesonephric duct is created when it "pinches off" the urogenital ridge to form a new tube. At the top end, the paramesonephric duct is in open communication with the abdominal cavity. This open end stays open and functions as the fimbriae of the uterine tubes. Towards the middle of the paramesonephric duct, fusion will occur with the paramesonephric duct on the other side. Only the lower portion fuses, the upper part remain as the uterine tubes. This fusion, and subsequent growth of tissue results in the development of the uterus and cervix. Eventually a muscular coating (myometrium) and a connective tissue coating (perimetrium) will form.

7.4.2 The Vagina

As the paramesonephric tubercle approaches the urogenital sinus, two growths called the sinovaginal bulbs appear. These bulbs form a piece of solid tissue and with continued growth, the cervix moves further away from the urogenital sinus. By week 20, the vagina has a canal that is separated from the urogenital sinus by the hymen.

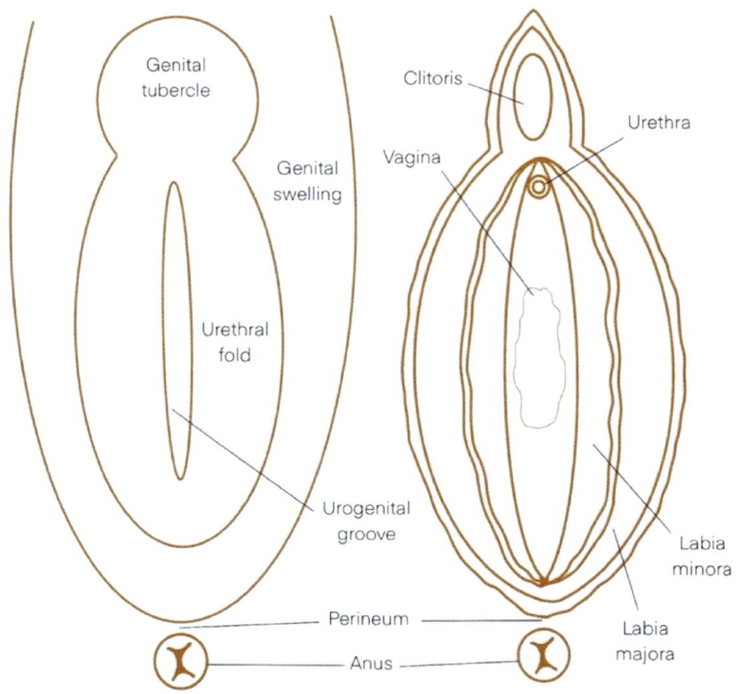

Image 7.6: Development of the external reproductive system.
Left: Week 20. Right: Birth.

The mesonephric duct almost completely vanishes in thin air except at the top and bottom ends. At the top end, the epoophoron is developed (equivalent to epididymis in male), and at the bottom end, the paroophoron (equivalent to paradidymis in male) is formed. Their function is unknown, but they may undergo pathological changes at some point in life (cysts and adenomas). Pathological variations of all topics will be described in Easy Embryology: Part 2.

7.4.3 The External Female Reproductive System

Oestrogen triggers development of the external components of the genitals in females. The genital tubercle only slightly elongates to form the clitoris, but unlike in the male the urethral folds do not fuse. Rather, they develop into the labia minora. The labia majora is derived from the genital swellings.

7.4.4 The Mammary Glands

Mammary glands (breast tissue) are discussed now, in this chapter, even though they probably should belong in the chapter that outlines the embryology of the skin. This is because the mammary glands are a customised sweat gland that is derived from ectoderm. They develop when the epidermis on each side of the embryo below the upper limbs thicken to form mammary ridges. The tissue of the mammary ridges then enters the mesoderm that is below it and forms multiple solid buds. These become the lactiferous ducts when the centre of these buds hollows out. The lactiferous buds will eventually drain out into the nipple.

Breast development is not complete at birth. Rather, during puberty, oestrogen, and progesterone production led to the formation of alveoli and the cells responsible for milk production. The breasts grow during puberty with varying outcomes between individuals.

Chapter 8: The Nervous System

In this chapter we will talk about the brain and spinal cord, and briefly discuss the peripheral nervous system. Chapter 8 is a long and difficult chapter, but this is relative to the other chapters. With that said, the simplification process itself has led to the omission of a lot of the minutiae in the development of the nervous system.

8.1 The Central Nervous System (CNS)

8.1.1 Development in General

A slight thickening of the ectoderm marks the humble beginning of the CNS. This thickened ectoderm is called the neural plate. When the edges of neural plate move up it is known as the neural folds. Eventually the neural folds "pinch off" the ectoderm in a way causing the edges to fuse together to form the neural tube. This process is called neurulation. This tube remains open at its top and bottom ends. These openings are called the cranial and caudal neuropores respectively. The cranial neuropore closes during week four and the caudal neuropore will close soon after. The top end of the neural tube becomes dilated in three separate areas, these are the primary brain vesicles. These vesicles are the forebrain, midbrain, and hindbrain. Memorise that the forebrain is the prosencephalon, the midbrain is the mesencephalon, and the hindbrain is the rhombencephalon prior to reading Section 8.1.3.

The location between the hindbrain and the rest of the neural tube (spinal cord) is called the cervical flexure. Another flexure, the cephalic flexure is located at the midbrain.

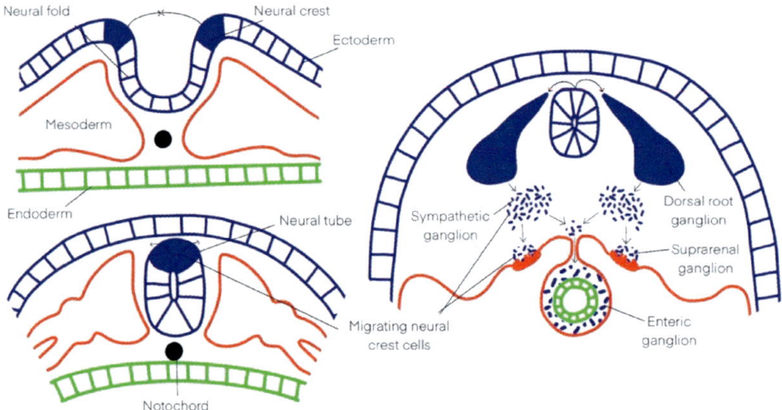

Image 8.1: Neurulation and the migration of neural crest cells.

Around week six the prosencephalon forms into the telencephalon and diencephalon. The mesencephalon is the midbrain, and the rhombencephalon forms into the metencephalon and myelencephalon. Between the metencephalon and myelencephalon is the pontine flexure. A lot of new words are being thrown at you in the same sentence but it's quite easy to understand if you memorise the words and associate them with Image 8.2.

Each brain vesicle has a cavity that corresponds to the future ventricle in which cerebrospinal fluid flows. The rhombencephalon's cavity is the fourth ventricle, the cavity of the diencephalon is the third ventricle and the cerebral cavities surround the lateral ventricles. The mesencephalon has the aqueduct of Sylvius which connects the third and fourth ventricles. The interventricular foramina of Monro is the communicating duct between the lateral ventricles and the third ventricle.

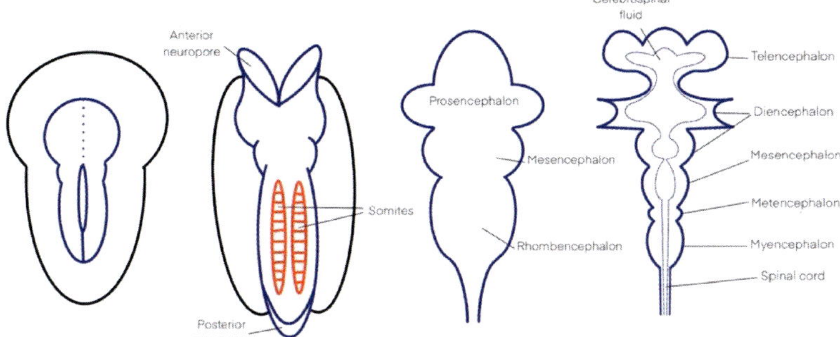

Image 8.2: The development of the CNS.

8.1.2 The Spinal Cord

The wall of the neural tube consists of neuroepithelial cells which together is termed the neuroepithelium. The neuroepithelium form neuroblasts (primitive nerve cells) which turn into the grey matter by forming a mantle layer surrounding the neuroepithelium. The white matter is developed from the marginal layer which is a layer made by the neuroblasts in the mantle layer. The white matter is white because they are myelinated.

High Yield!

The spinal cord extends only to the level of L2/L3 and the nerves that continue past this point are known as the cauda equina.

The mantle layer continues to grow and produces a ventral and a dorsal growth on either side. The ventral growths are called the basal plates and consist of the ventral motor horn cells. The dorsal growths are called alar plates and form the dorsal sensory horn cells. You can remember alar being associated with sensory by thinking of an alarm being so loud that it activates your senses, and therefore basal is motor by elimination.

8.1.3 The Brain

This section will describe the development of the brain from the cortex all the way down the brain stem. It is quite a complicated process, therefore there is a lot of information to digest. Despite simplification in our usual manner, there are a lot of new words to learn. Go through it slowly, visualise the processes with the images, and you'll understand. We break down the embryology of the brain into three parts: forebrain, midbrain, and hindbrain.

8.1.3.1 The Forebrain

The forebrain, known as the prosencephalon, forms the telencephalon and the diencephalon.

Telencephalon

The telencephalon develops into the cerebral hemispheres as two lateral growths and one medial growth at the end of the first month of development. The medial growth is called the lamina terminalis. At week seven, the lower end of the developing cerebral hemispheres proliferates and pushes into the ventricles. This is the developing corpus striatum. It continues to grow and divides into the caudate nucleus and the lentiform nucleus. The cerebrum continues to grow anteriorly to form the frontal lobes, dorsally to form the temporal lobes and inferiorly to form the occipital lobes. The insula remains deep to these lobes as its growth is relatively slow.

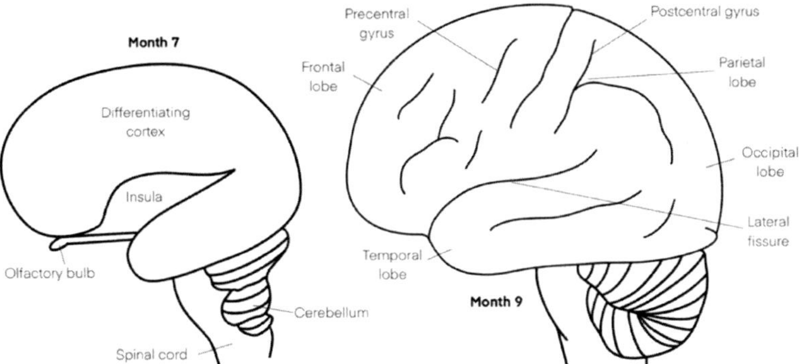

Image 8.3: Cortex differentiation into distinct lobes.

A bunch of nerves known as commissures connect the left and right cerebral hemispheres. Three commissures are derived from the lamina terminalis. Connecting the olfactory bulb with its important relations is the anterior commissure. The corpus callosum connects most of the other parts of one hemisphere to the relevant structure on the other side. Finally, the hippocampal commissure connects the hippocampus to the hypothalamus and mammillary body. The part of the telencephalon that meets with the diencephalon will form the choroid plexus.

Diencephalon

The diencephalon develops into the pituitary, thalamus, hypothalamus, pineal body, and the optic cup/stalk system and is made up from a roof plate and two alar plates. The roof plates develop into a choroid plexus that secrete cerebrospinal fluid into the third ventricle. The lower end of the roof plate will become the pineal body. The hypothalamic sulcus will divide the alar plates into the thalamus and the hypothalamus.

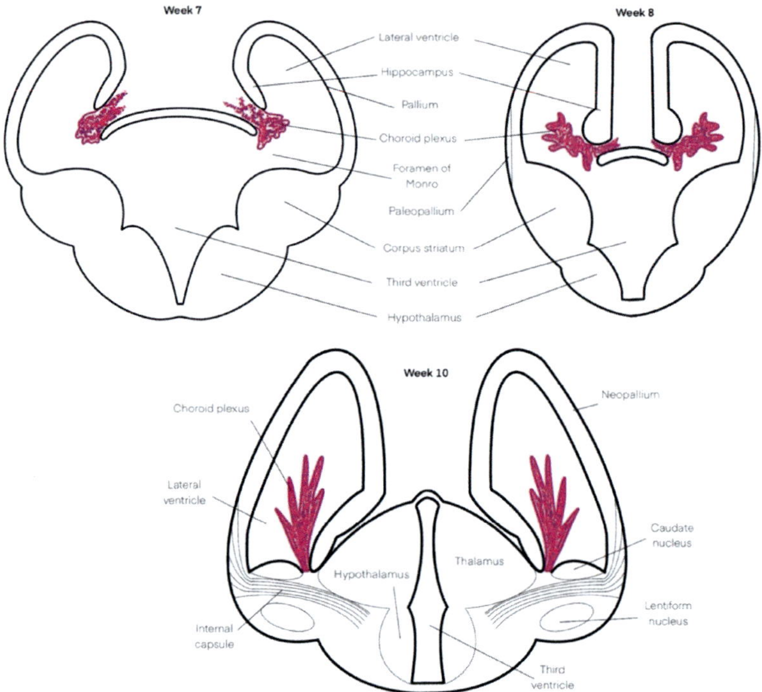

Image 8.4: Development of the forebrain. Cross-sections through the prosencephalon.

The pituitary gland comes from the ectoderm of the stomodeum as well as from the infundibulum which is a growth from the diencephalon. The stomodeum is the primitive mouth (think of the stomodeum as the opening to the stomach and duodenum). Rathke's pouch begins developing from the oral cavity at three weeks. It grows towards the infundibulum and becomes its neighbour after detaching from the oral cavity. Cells in the anterior portion of Rathke's pouch will form the anterior pituitary lobe (adenohypophysis). The posterior portion of Rathke's pouch does not amount to anything worth discussing.

8.1.3.2 The Midbrain

The mesencephalon contains two motor groups in its basal plate. There is a medial (somatic) and a lateral motor group (called the nucleus of Edinger-Westphal). The medial contains the oculomotor and trochlear cranial nerves (motor). The lateral contains fibres that control the sphincter pupillary muscle. The marginal layer of the basal plates develops into the crus cerebri.

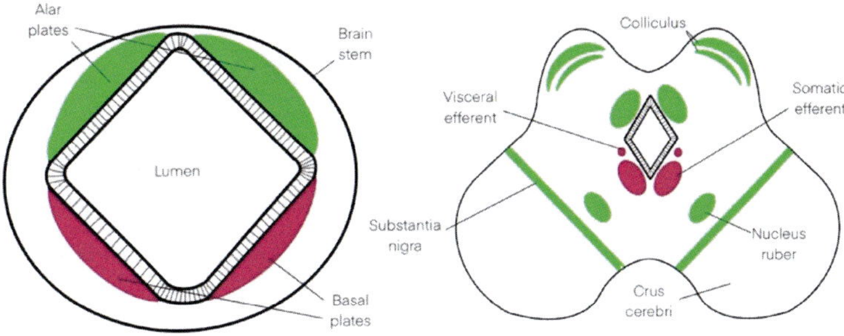

Image 8.5: Cross-sections through the mesencephalon at two different points in time.

The alar plates develop into the anterior and posterior colliculus (sensory). The anterior colliculus allows for reflexes in response to visual stimuli, and the posterior for auditory stimuli. For example, if you are surprised by a large bang from a door slamming you might jump in fright, this reflex uses the posterior colliculus as a relay.

8.1.3.3 The Hindbrain

The rhombencephalon consists of the myelencephalon and the metencephalon. The myelencephalon becomes the medulla oblongata, whereas the metencephalon forms the cerebellum and the pons. The pons contains nerves that acts as a messenger system between the cerebellum, cerebrum and spinal cord.

Metencephalon

The basal plates of the metencephalon contain a similar structure of motor nuclei to the myelencephalon. Its medial group develops the nucleus of the abducens nerve, the intermediate houses the nucleus of the facial and trigeminal cranial nerves, and the lateral group supplies the submandibular and sublingual glands. The trigeminal cranial nerve is also contributed to by the alar plates.

The rhombic lips of the cerebellum are formed once the alar plates of the metencephalon begin to bend towards the middle. These lips develop to form the cerebellar plate and at the third month, this plate differentiates to form the vermis at the midline and two lateral hemispheres. The nodule is developed from the vermis and separates the flocculus, which is developed from the lateral hemispheres. This is how the flocculonodular lobe is developed. It is the earliest form of the cerebellum. The neuroepithelium produce cells that will form the granular layer and these cells continue to divide on the surface of the cerebellum giving rise to all the different types of cells of the cerebellum by week 24.

Myelencephalon

The basal plate of the myelencephalon contains three groups of motor nuclei. These are a medial, intermediate and a lateral. The medial group supplies somatic nerves. These are the hypoglossal, abducens, trochlear and oculomotor cranial nerves. The intermediate group contains special visceral nerves. These include the accessory, vagus and glossopharyngeal cranial nerves. The lateral group supplies the muscles that are not under voluntary control (breathing, peristalsis, heart beating and studying).

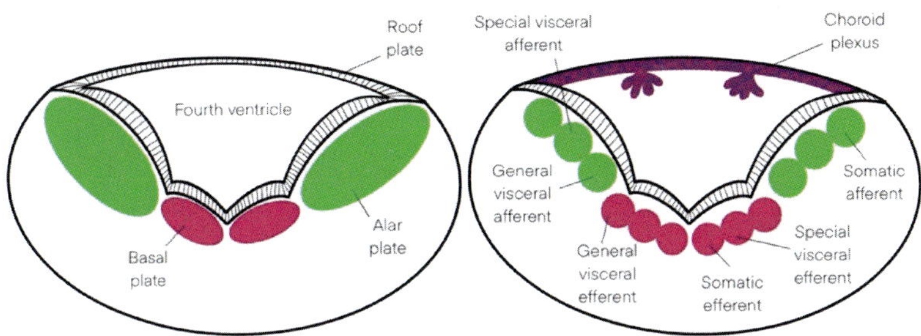

Image 8.6: The basal and alar plates of the myelencephalon differentiating into their subsequent important structures.

The alar plate also contains three groups of sensory nuclei. Again, a medial, intermediate, and a lateral. The lateral gets information about pain, temperature and touch via the glossopharyngeal nerve. The intermediate gets taste, sound, and balance information from the vestibulocochlear nerve; and the medial gets information from the heart and the gut.

8.1.3.4 The Cranial Nerves

Cranial nerves I and II come from the telencephalon, and III is from the mesencephalon. In the rhombencephalon, eight segments called the rhombomeres develop. These are the centres that the other eight cranial nerves (V – XII) develop. The cranial nerves with sensory ganglia are located on the outside of the brainstem, whereas the cranial nerves with motor neurons are contained inside the brainstem. The sensory ganglia come from ectodermal placodes as well as neural crest cells. The ectodermal placodes are thickenings the ectoderm. The placodes include the nasal, otic, and four pairs of epibrachial placodes. The parasympathetic fibres of cranial nerves III, VII, IX, and X are developed from the neural crest cells.

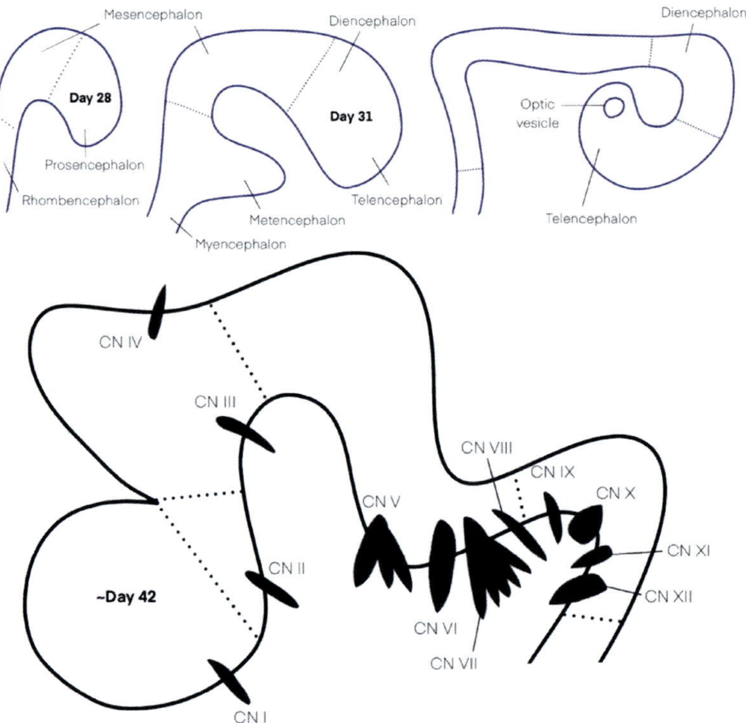

Image 8.7: The cranial nerves and development of the brain throughout various stages.

8.2 The Peripheral Nervous System (PNS)

8.2.1 The Sympathetic Nervous System

Neural crest cells move from the lateral sides of the spinal cord to behind the dorsal aorta in the second month (Image 8.1). In this region, the neural crest cells form the sympathetic ganglia that are all in communication with each other by long nerves. These are the trunks of the sympathetic nervous system. Neuroblasts help in lengthening the sympathetic nervous system from top to bottom. They also develop into the celiac and mesenteric ganglia, and the sympathetic organ plexuses in the heart, lungs and the gastrointestinal tract. The lateral horns of the spinal column at T1-L3 connect with the sympathetic ganglia to become the fibres which stimulate the sympathetic nerves. These nerves have myelin and are therefore white (white communicating rami). The postganglionic fibres have no myelin. The grey communicating rami go from the sympathetic trunk to the nerves in the spine and then to the blood vessels, sweat glands, and hair (think of the fight or flight response when the sympathetic nervous system is activated).

8.2.2 Parasympathetic nervous system

Neural crest cells also form the ganglia of the parasympathetic system. Parasympathetic preganglionic neurons develop their nuclei in the locations of cranial nerves III, VII, IX, and X as well as in the S2-S4 region. To know what organs they innervate, work it out yourself by thinking about how it is also called the "rest and digest" system.

Chapter 9: Head and Neck

The pharyngeal arches (some ancient texts describe them as brachial arches) are central in the formation of the head, face, and neck and are what make the embryo initially look like an alien. The pharyngeal arches begin development at the end of the first month. Development of the pharyngeal arches, which is described in Section 9.1, is closely linked to the pharyngeal clefts, and pharyngeal pouches that are subsequently described in Sections 9.2 and 9.3. The clefts are formed from the bulging of the arches which are at first slabs of tissue. The clefts are external to the embryo, whereas the pouches are internal (Image 9.1). Think of the clefts as being cliffs, which are on the outside, and pouches as a kangaroo pouch, the joey relaxing on the inside. Needed at least one Australian reference in this book.

9.1 The Pharyngeal Arches

A pharyngeal arch is made of a mesoderm centre, specifically a paraxial and lateral plate mesoderm centre. It is coated with ectoderm and neural crest cells on the outside, and its insides are layered with endoderm, which contributes to its epithelial layer. Even though there are five pairs of arches in total, there is no fifth arch. That is, the arches are labelled from I, II, III, IV, and VI – no V. This is because arch V does not contribute to anything, disappearing into another dimension. Each arch has its own specific cranial nerve and blood supply that is conveniently summarised in Image 9.2.

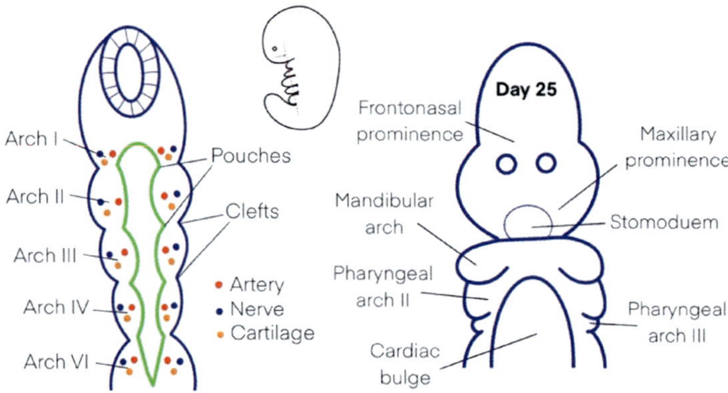

Image 9.1: A section through the embryo at the level of the pharyngeal arches. Demonstrates how each arch has its own artery, cranial nerve, and cartilage. The green lining is endoderm.

The best way to learn the embryology of the pharyngeal arches is to look at Image 9.2 and memorise what each arch becomes. When memorising, if you visualise the diagrams (Image 9.3) it's easier to remember. Forget about a mnemonic to memorise this. The best way to remember is to visualise and understand. Otherwise during the exam, you might remember the mnemonic but not what it stands for.

Arch I is made up from a maxillary and a mandibular process. Meckel's cartilage is a part of the first pharyngeal arch (mandibular part) and will eventually form the incus and malleus. A summary of what the rest of the arches develop into is shown in Image 9.2.

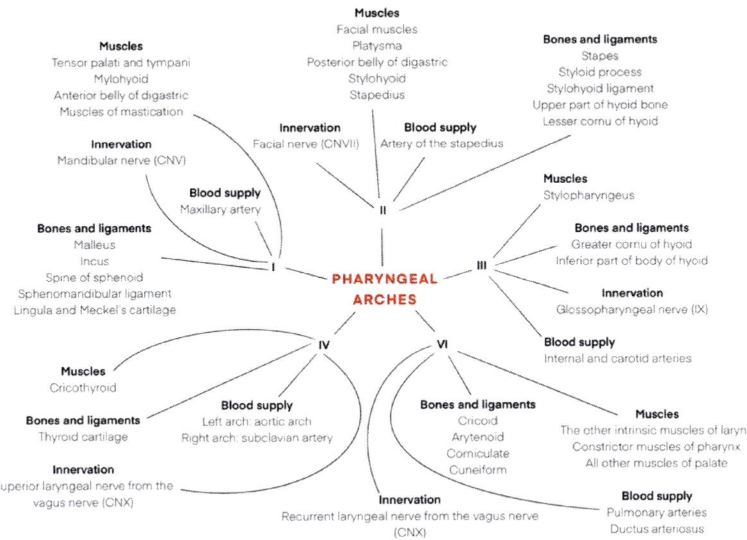

Image 9.2: What each pharyngeal arch contributes to in terms of final structures of the head and neck.

9.2 The Pharyngeal Pouches

There are four sets of pharyngeal pouches. Again, there is no fifth pouch – it is only a temporary structure that does not contribute to anything known. Remember, the pouches are on the inside, so they are derived from mostly endoderm. The pouches each contribute to high yield structures in the adult as described below.

Pouch I forms the tubotympanic recess, which continues to grow outward until it comes into contact with the epithelium from first pharyngeal cleft. The most external part of the tubotympanic recess will become the middle ear, and the point where Pouch I meets Cleft I becomes the tympanic membrane. The most internal part of the tubotympanic recess will become the internal auditory tube. This tube links the nasopharynx to the middle ear.

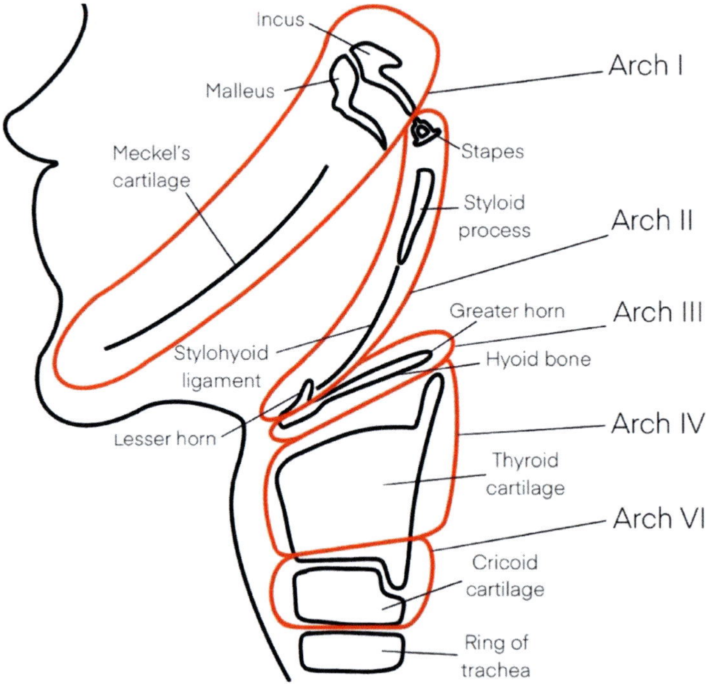

Image 9.3: Use this image in conjunction with Image 9.2 to help visualise what each pharyngeal arch contributes to.

The Pouch II epithelium proliferates and penetrates the mesoderm surrounding it to form the palatine tonsils.

Having a dorsal and ventral component seems to be a recurring theme in embryology. Pouch III is not the exception. Pouch III also has a dorsal and a ventral component. The dorsal part becomes the inferior parathyroid gland. Initially, the inferior parathyroid gland is above the superior parathyroid gland which is derived from pouch IV.

However, they lose connection with their surrounding walls and move down into their final position behind the thyroid gland unless it turns out to be an ectopic (in which case good luck finding it). The superior parathyroid gland also moves down, but the inferior parathyroid glands move down further. Due to the longer distance travelled to reach their final position, the locations of the inferior parathyroid glands are more variable. The ventral part of pouch III becomes the thymus. The thymus also detaches from the wall and moves down. The ventral components of each pouch III will fuse on their downward movement becoming a single thymus gland.

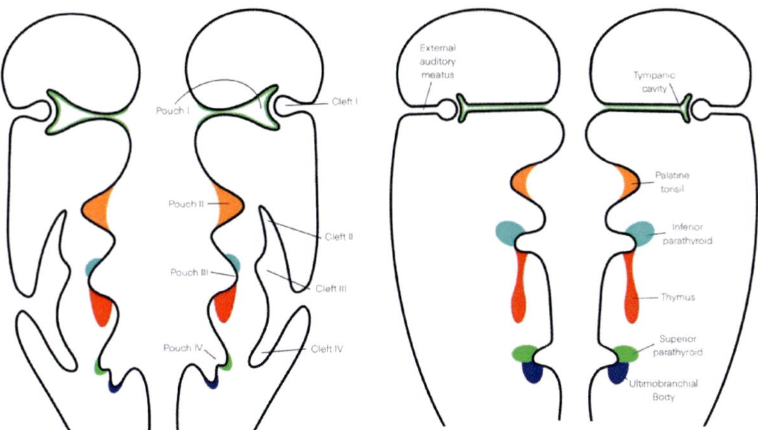

Image 9.4: The development of the pharyngeal pouches. Very important structures are derived, such as the parathyroid glands. See Image 9.5 for the next step.

Pouch IV happens to also have a dorsal and ventral component. The dorsal part becomes the superior parathyroid gland. As the inferior parathyroid gland rides on the coattails of the thymus gland on its descent, the superior thyroid glands jump onto the descending thyroid gland. The dorsal part of pouch IV develops into the C cells (parafollicular cells) of the thyroid.

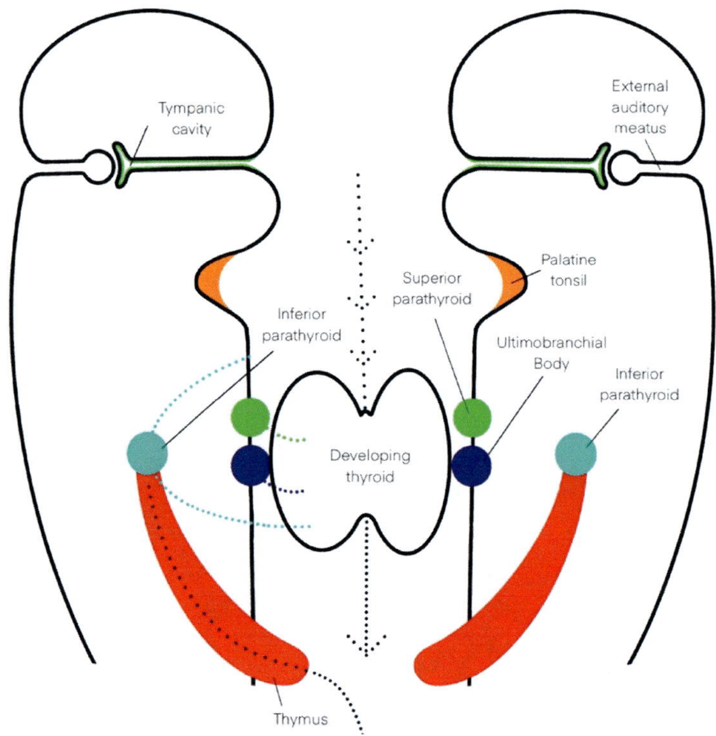

Image 9.5: This image demonstrates the relationship of the structures of the pharyngeal pouches to the descending and developing thyroid.

9.3 The Pharyngeal Clefts

There are four pairs of pharyngeal clefts, however only the first cleft contributes to anything worthwhile. We also touched on this when discussing the first pouch – the external auditory meatus. The rest of the clefts are temporary structures and completely disappear as the arches continue to develop.

9.4 The Tongue

At week four, three swellings from the first pharyngeal arch pop-out. The growths are the two lateral lingual swellings and one medial lingual swelling which is called the tuberculum impar. Pharyngeal arches II, III, and IV contribute to another medial swelling called the copula. Arch IV also contributes to another medial swelling which will become the epiglottis, and another opportunity will be taken to mention that pharyngeal arch V does nothing. The lateral lingual swellings eventually fuse together to form the anterior 2/3 of the tongue.

Keep in mind that the innervation of nerves to various parts of the tongue depend on which pharyngeal arch they come from. Thus, sensory innervation of the anterior 2/3 of the tongue is supplied by the mandibular component of the trigeminal nerve. Arch IV contributes to the posterior 1/3 of the tongue and thus sensory innervation is via the glossopharyngeal nerve. The glossopharyngeal nerve also innervates the sense of taste for the posterior 1/3. On the other hand, the sense of taste of the anterior 2/3 is supplied by the chorda tympani branch of the facial nerve. The muscle of the tongue is innervated by the hypoglossal nerve.

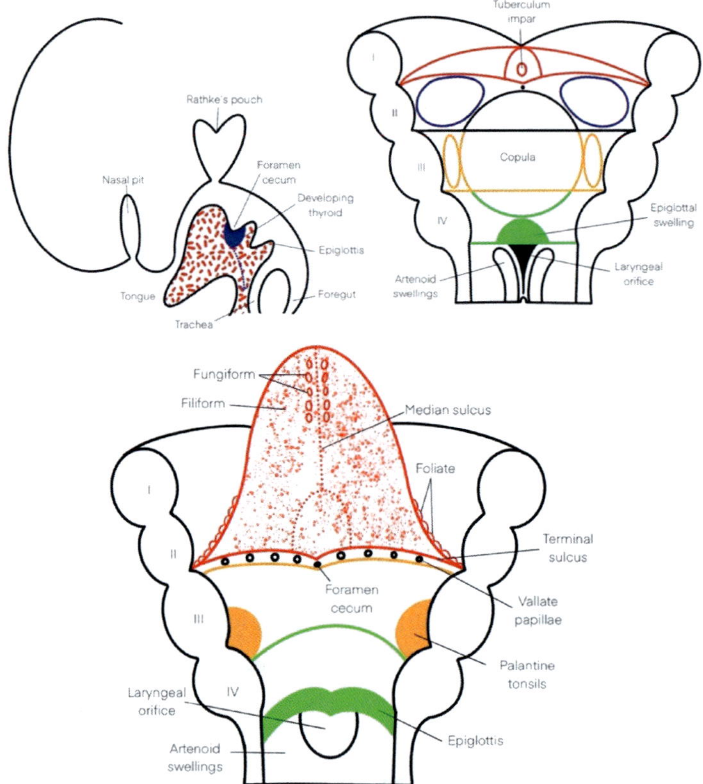

Image 9.6: The development of the tongue drawn relative to the pharyngeal arches.

9.5 The Thyroid

The development of the thyroid gland is discussed in this chapter due to proximity to the aforementioned structures. Given we have just discussed the parathyroid glands and the other important structures derived from the pharyngeal arches and pouches, learning the development of the thyroid gland in this context will allow for a more holistic understanding.

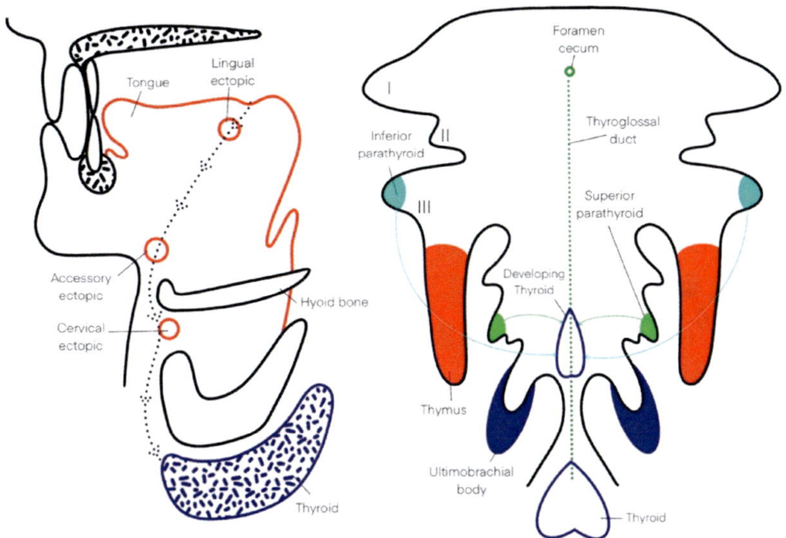

Image 9.7: The descent of the thyroid. The coloured lines show each structure's path.

The thyroid is born from the epithelium of the pharynx between the tuberculum impar and the copula (the swellings of the tongue). Thus, the thyroid gland is born from endoderm. The thyroid descends and will continue to grow on its descent until it has formed two lobes, all the while remaining attached to the tongue by the thyroglossal duct. The final position of the thyroid will be in front of the trachea, reaching this location by the end of month two. At this point the thyroid has grown two full lobes, an isthmus, and a pyramidal lobe in 10% of the population.

9.6 The Face

By the second month, the facial prominences begin to develop from the first pharyngeal arch and the neural crest cells. The maxillary prominences are found on either side of the developing mouth (the stomodeum). The mandibular prominence is found below the mouth and the frontonasal prominence is above it. The nasal placodes are on either side of the frontonasal prominence and they form the nasal pits. Surrounding each pit are the nasal prominences, a lateral and a medial nasal prominence.

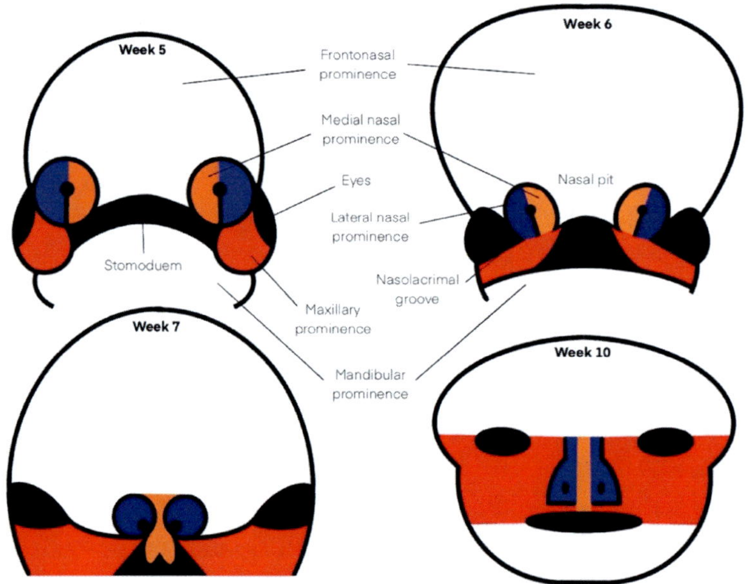

Image 9.8: The development of the face. Colour coded throughout weeks 5 to 10 according to each prominence.

The maxillary prominences grow and push the medial nasal prominences towards the middle and they fuse together. The upper lip is formed from both medial nasal prominences and both maxillary prominences. The lower lip and jaw are from the mandibular prominences. The nose is formed from all five facial prominences. Frontal forms the bridge, the crest and tip from the medial, and the alae is from the lateral.

The nasal prominences also fuse at a deeper level to form the intermaxillary segment. There is a labial part which forms the philtrum, an upper jaw part that comprise of the four incisors, and a palatal part forming the primary palate. The maxillary prominences form palatine shelves which fuse above the tongue to form the secondary palate (Image 9.10). The secondary palate fuses with the primary palate, the midline of which is called the incisive foramen.

The nasal pits become deeper and the oronasal membrane that separates the pits from the oral cavity disintegrates. The paranasal air sinuses develop from the wall of the nasal cavity by spreading into the maxilla, ethmoid, sphenoid, and frontal bones of the skull. The growth of these sinuses contributes to the shape of the person's face especially following puberty. The shape is also obviously contributed by the mandible and the maxilla.

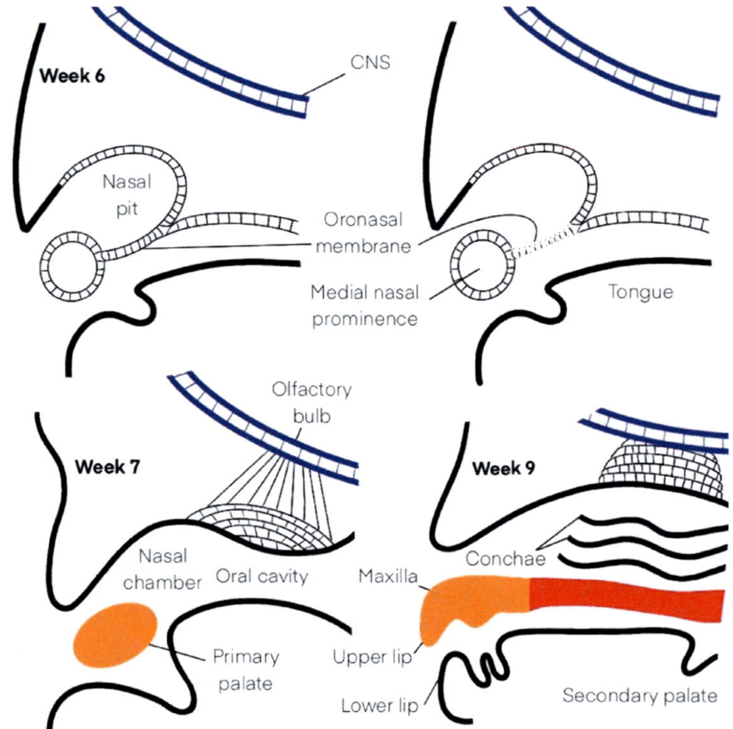

Image 9.9: Fusion of the primary and secondary plate and partitioning of the nasal and oral cavities.

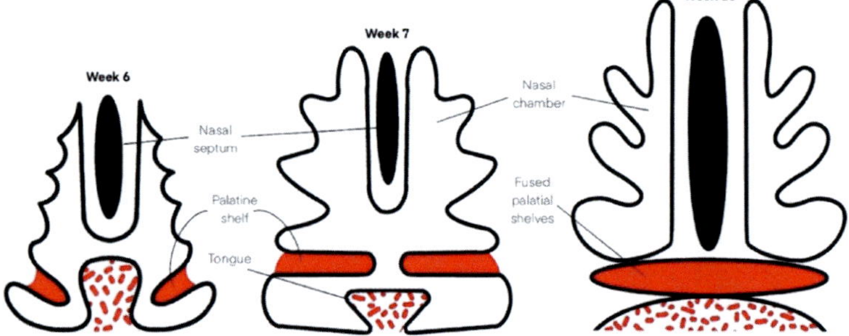

Image 9.10: Frontal-sections demonstrating how the fusion of the palatine shelves separate the oral cavity from the nasal cavity.

Chapter 10: The Eyes

Development of the eye is slightly more complex than most of the organs already discussed, but if you need to know the embryology of the eyes, then you are probably training to be an ophthalmologist. This is the life you chose.

The eye is first seen around week three. Just like the development of ears are first heard of once an otic placode appears and then turns into an otic vesicle (Chapter 11), the eyes similarly first appear in the form of an optic placode and turns into an optic vesicle. The optic placodes, which is born out of the neural tube, will develop into the optic vesicles. Thus, the eye is derived from ectoderm.

The optic vesicles grow until they touch the 'skin' of the embryo. The lens then forms, and the optic vesicle forms the optic cup. The optic cup has two layers: an inner and an outer layer. The outer layer is the pigmented layer of the retina, and the inner layer is the neural layer. In week seven, the optic cup begins to form the pupil. The actual lens itself is developed from the ectoderm as a lens placode, and by week five it lets go of the ectoderm and moves to the optic cup.

The pars optica retinae is the outermost layer of the inner layer and will contain the rods and cones. Next to the pars optica retinae is the mantle layer which develops into the neurons of the eye (outer nuclear, inner nuclear, and ganglion layers). The axons of these nerves are on the surface, and they will form the optic nerve (CNII). The most anterior part of the inner layer has a one cell coating, called the pars ceca retinae, which will form both the pars iridica retinae (the inner layer of the iris) and the pars ciliaris retinae (which becomes the ciliary body). The pars ciliaris retinae continually folds to give it its squiggly appearance and the ciliary muscle will eventually control the lens in response to light and other exciting stimuli. The dilator pupillae and the sphincter of the eye form in the epithelial cells contained within the surface and the optic cup.

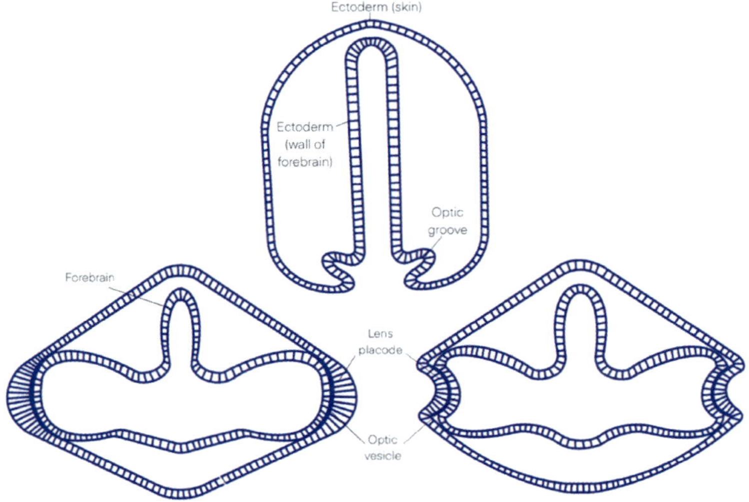

Image 10.1: Cross sections of the forebrain at the level of the developing eye. Top: The day 22 embryo showing the optic groove in relation to the forebrain. Left: The day 28 embryo showing contact between the lens placode and optic vesicle. Right: Both the lens placode and optic vesicle begin to "pinch off" the ectoderm. Lots of pinching occurs in this book.

There is another inner and outer layer for you to remember now, because the tissue that surrounds the eye will also form an inner and outer layer. The inner layer will become a tissue similar to the pia mater, and the outer layer the dura mater. The pia mater portion becomes the choroid, and the dura mater portion becomes the sclera.

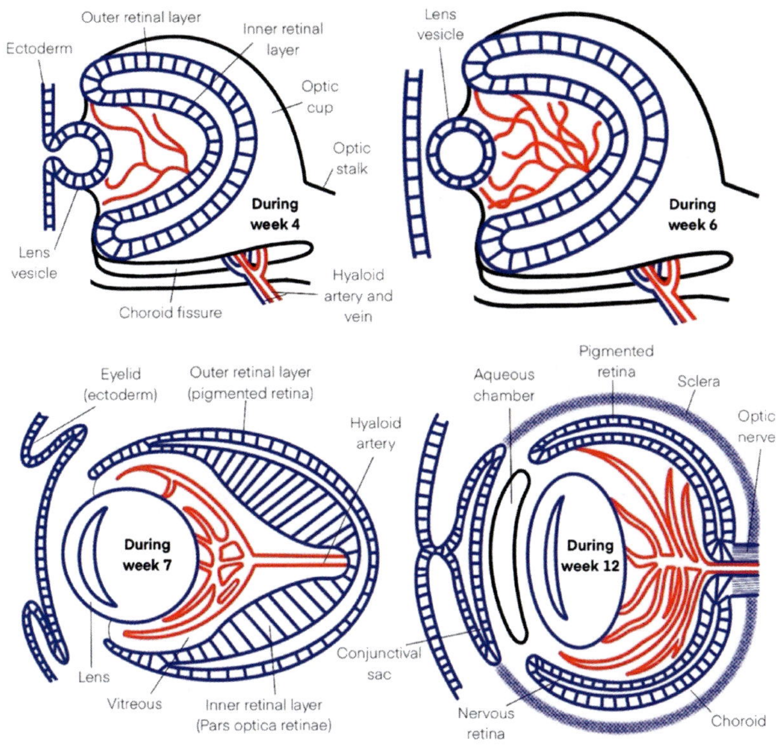

Image 10.2: Cross-sections of the developing eye between weeks 4 and 12.

The anterior chamber of the eye forms when there is degeneration of tissue that yet again forms an inner and outer layer. The inner layer is the iridopupillary membrane (which disappears anterior to the lens) and the outer layer is the substantia propria. The cornea is made from the substantia propria, an epithelial layer from ectoderm, and the epithelium shared with the anterior chamber. The posterior chamber is surrounded by the iris and ciliary body. Both anterior and posterior chambers are in open communication with each other through the pupil, and both contain aqueous humor that perpetually circulates.

Between the retina and the lens, the vitreous body is created by migrating tissue that was previously surrounding the optic cup.

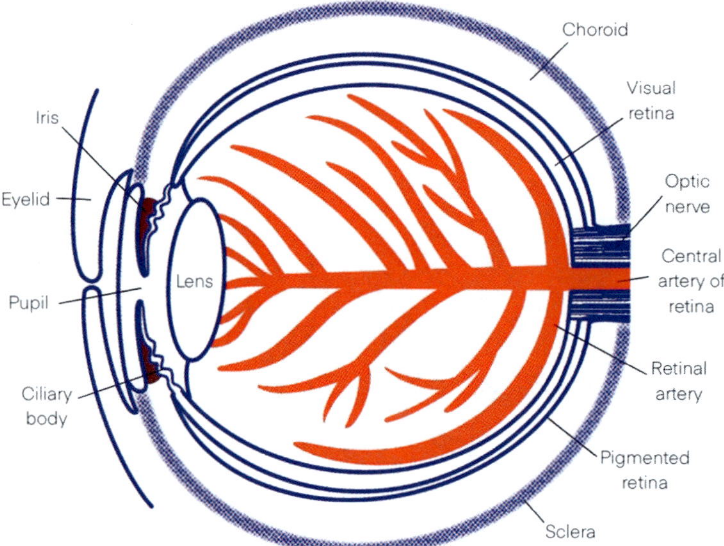

Image 10.3: The eye at week 30.

Chapter 11: The Ear

The ear has three parts to it. These are the inner, middle and external. We will discuss their embryology in three separate sections.

11.1 The Inner Ear

The ear begins developing by week three. The growth of the otic placodes on the ectoderm is the first appearance of the ear. This occurs near the level of the hindbrain on both sides. The placodes transform into otic vesicles when they start digging into the embryo and pinching off the ectoderm (Image 11.1). The vesicles then evolve into a ventral and a dorsal part. The ventral part will develop into the saccule and cochlear duct. The dorsal part will become the utricle, semicircular canals, and the endolymph duct (Image 11.2). Thus, the otic vesicles begot the membranous labyrinth.

A growth from the saccule is called the cochlear duct. It will spiral for three long weeks until it reaches two-and-a-half turns. It is complete in a normal scenario by the end of the second month. The scala vestibuli and scala tympani are the two perilymphatic spaces that are formed when cartilage surrounding the cochlear duct becomes hollow. The vestibular membrane separates the scala vestibuli from the cochlear duct, and the basilar membrane separates the scala tympani from the cochlear duct (Image 11.3).

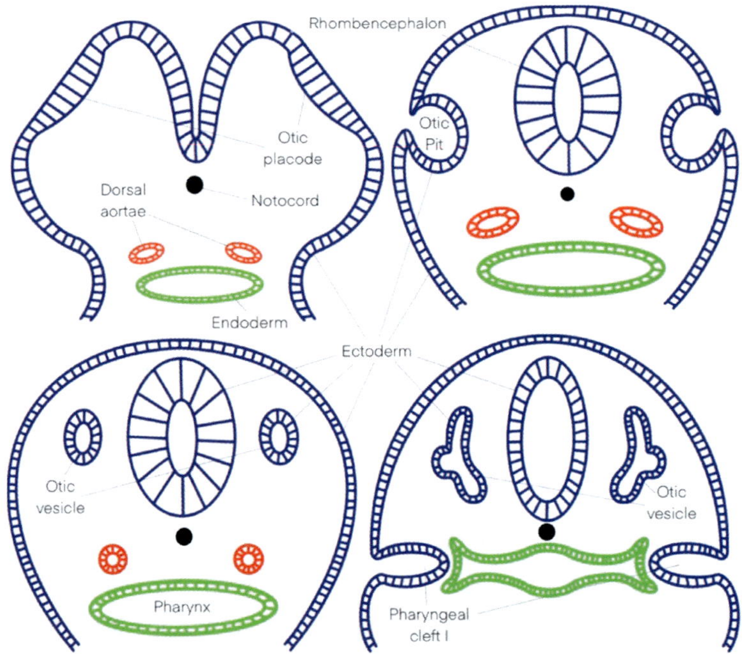

Image 11.1: The development of the inner ear represented by formation of otic vesicles. This image demonstrates the thickening of ectoderm in week 3 (top-left), until it pinches off and differentiates into the utricle and saccule (bottom-right).

Now let's discuss the inner part of the inner ear. Inside the cochlear duct, the epithelium differentiates into an inner ridge and an outer ridge that forms the spiral limbus and the hair cells respectively. The hair cells are covered by the tectorial membrane which is also connected to the spiral limbus. The hair cells and the tectorial membrane are called the organ of Corti.

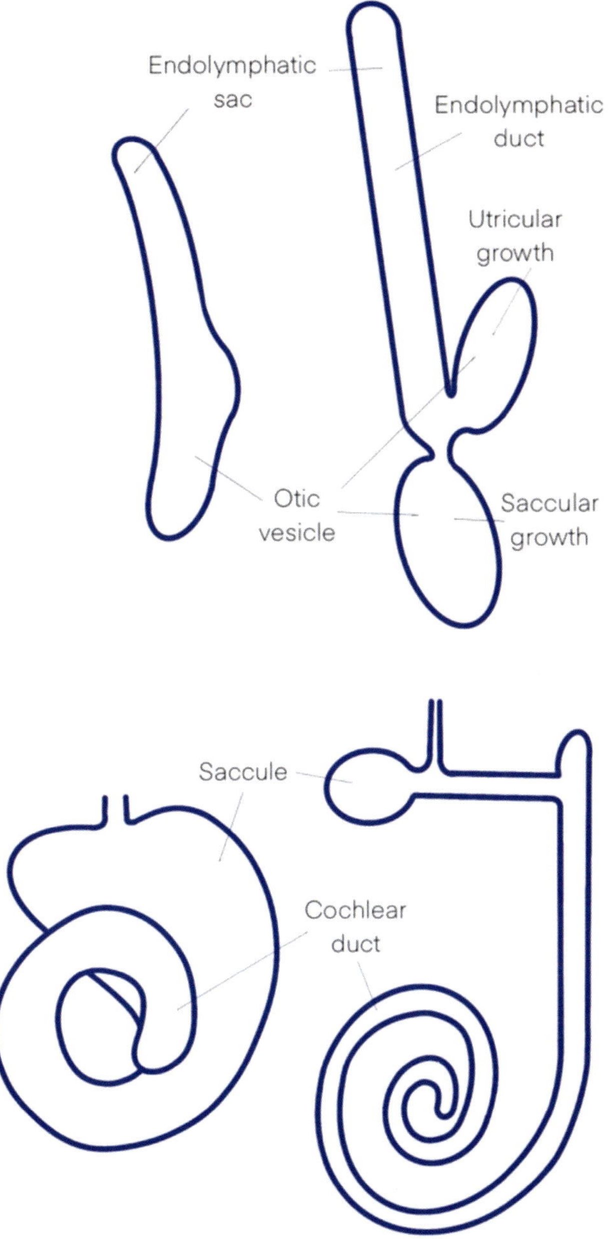

Image 11.2: The otic vesicle differentiates into the saccule and utricle.

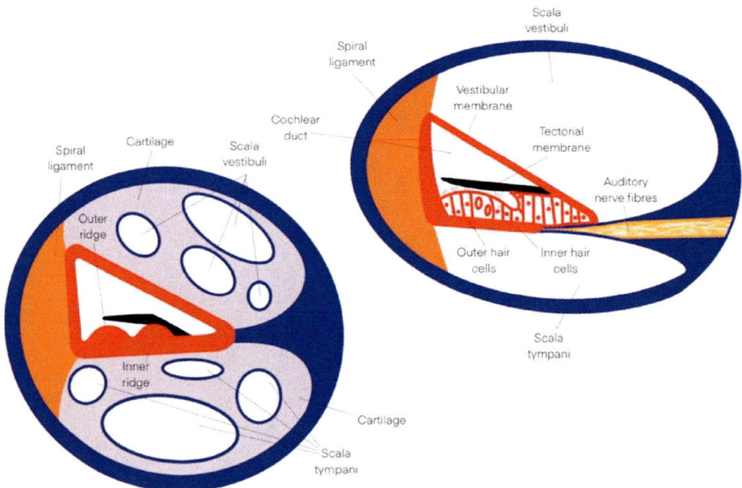

Image 11.3: Cross-sections of the cochlear duct. The cartilage (grey) degenerates making space for the scala vestibuli and the scala tympani.

High Yield!

Cells from the otic vesicle, which have their beginnings in the neural crest cell, will form a ganglion called the statoacoustic ganglion. This divides into both a vestibular component that innervates the saccule, utricle and semicircular canals, and a cochlear component that innervates the organ of Corti.

The semicircular canals appear approximately around day 42, growing out of the otic vesicle until three semicircular canals are formed. One end of the semicircular canal widens into an "ampule" (the crus ampullare) whereas the other end doesn't (the crus nonampullare). The cells in the crus ampullare become the sensory cells of balance that carry information to the vestibulocochlear nerve (cranial nerve VIII).

11.2 The Middle Ear

The endoderm contributes to the creation of the tympanic cavity. To understand this process, it may be a good idea to first learn about the embryology of the pharyngeal clefts and pouches (Chapter 9). However, if you're in a rush because your exam is in three minutes and you don't have the time, here is a brief repetition of that description. Pouch I grows towards the outside until it touches the first pharyngeal cleft. The most outer part of the first pharyngeal pouch becomes larger and becomes the primitive tympanic cavity, whereas the middle part remains thin to form the auditory tube.

The malleus, incus, and stapes are all developed from the pharyngeal arches. The malleus and incus develop from the first arch, and the stapes from the second. The bones are trapped within tissue as opposed to being surrounded by air, despite being developed by the eighth month. Eventually the tissue disappears to make the middle ear cavity larger. Then, the epithelium of the tympanic cavity grows to connect the bones to the walls of the cavity, holding them in place. Innervation of the structures are by the innervation of the pharyngeal arches in which they were born. That is, the tensor tympani (muscle of the malleus) is innervated by the trigeminal nerve (mandibular branch); and the muscle of the stapes, the stapedius, is innervated by the facial nerve. The developing epithelium of the tympanic cavity spreads into the mastoid process to form the air sacs in a process called pneumatisation.

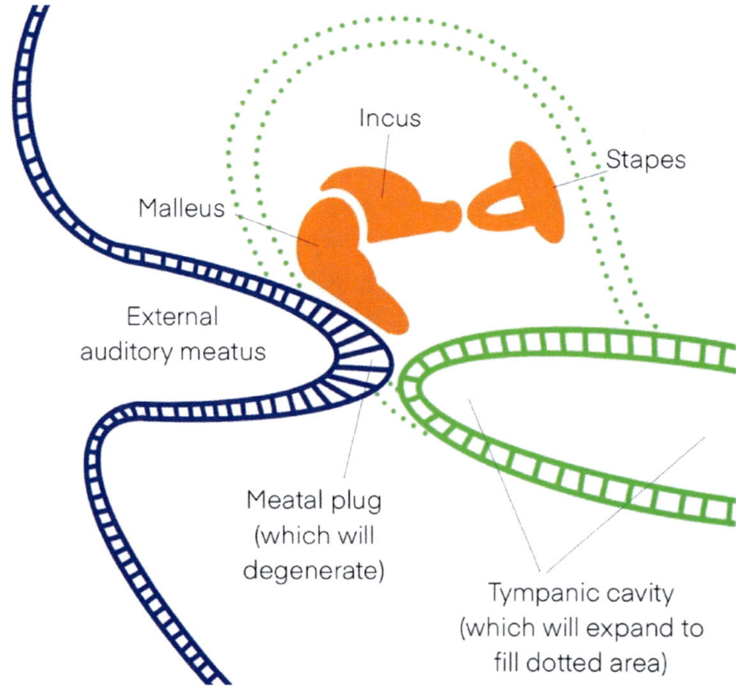

Image 11.4: The development of the middle ear. The tympanic cavity will expand until it surrounds the ear bones with air.

11.3 The External Ear

The external auditory canal is formed by the first pharyngeal cleft (Chapter 9). During week 12 the epithelium of the first pharyngeal cleft is a solid tissue. However, this tissue eventually mostly disappears leaving behind a single sheet of epithelium which contributes to the tympanic membrane. The tympanic membrane is made from endoderm, ectoderm and mesoderm. In the same order as described in Chapter 1. The ectoderm is on the outside. It is continuous with the epithelium of the external ear. The mesoderm consists of the middle fibrous layer; and the endoderm makes the inner layer and is continuous with the inner ear epithelium.

Even more external than the external auditory meatus is the auricle. It is the floppy part of the external ear that everyone can see, touch, and some can even wiggle. It develops from pharyngeal arches I and II. The auricular hillocks are six individual growths from the first two pharyngeal arches (three on each side). As the mandible grows, it pulls the auricle up with it from the neck to the level of the eyes and all three components fuse to form the final form of the ear.

Chapter 12: The Teeth

The teeth develop from the oral epithelium and its underlying tissue which is made from the neural crest cells. The oral epithelium forms the dental lamina along the jaws which develops to form ten dental buds in each upper and lower jaw.

These buds bury themselves inwards marking the beginning of the cap stage. The cap is now made up of an outer and inner dental epithelium, and an inner core called the stellate reticulum. The bell stage of tooth development is when the tooth grows so much it starts to look like a bell. Dentin secreting odontoblasts are derived from dental papilla cells closest to the inner dental later. The rest of the papilla form the tooth's pulp which will form a canal to contain the blood vessels and nerves.

Ameloblasts that form the tooths enamel come from the inner dental epithelium, and the enamel is laid over the dentin beginning at the top which spreads and becomes thick. The ameloblasts move into the stellate reticulum leaving only the dental cuticle covering the enamel. The dental cuticle sloughs off the tooth once it grows out of the gums roughly two years after the baby is born.

Tissue surrounding the dentin near the root become cementoblasts that do as their name suggests, produce cementum. Holding the tooth in place is the periodontal ligament which also absorbs shock.

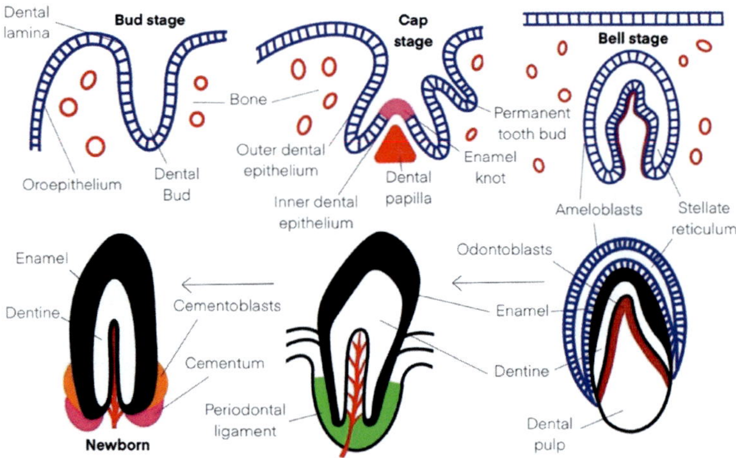

Image 12.1: The development of the teeth. Note that each image represents changes all occuring below the gums.

High Yield!

The permanent teeth which replace the milk teeth begin to develop at around week 12 but do not appear until six years of age. When they grow, they push out the milk teeth and replace them. Osteoclasts eat up the remaining root of the milk tooth.

Chapter 13: The Diaphragm

The diaphragm is made from muscle and tendon. It is developed from four important structures that will eventually separate the peritoneal cavity and the thoracic cavity. Prior to diaphragm development, the thoracic and peritoneal cavities are in open communication. That is, they are a single cavity. The four important structures are the septum transversum, the pleuroperitoneal membrane, the dorsal oesophageal membrane, and the actual body wall.

The septum transversum is a plate formed from the splanchnic mesoderm that will eventually separate the thoracic and abdominal cavities. It will become the central tendon of the diaphragm. It joins with tissue below the oesophagus and with the pleuroperitoneal membranes.

The open area at the level of the septum transversum is called the pericardioperitoneal canal. The pleuroperitoneal folds (appears in week four and survives until week six) grow towards the middle and to the front of the body to fuse with the mesentery of the oesophagus. At this point the pleural cavity and the peritoneal cavity are partitioned. The pleuroperitoneal folds also grow into the pleuropericardial membranes forming the fibrous layer of the pericardium. The dorsal oesophageal mesentery will make up the crura of the diaphragm.

As the foetus grows, the walls of the body also become larger. At week nine the pleural cavity continues to become larger and fuses with the walls of the body over the next four weeks. The tissue of the body walls then form the outermost portion of the diaphragm, the part that the pleuroperitoneal membranes failed to contribute to.

Eventually myoblasts from mesoderm penetrate the pleuroperitoneal membranes to form the muscular part of the diaphragm.

High Yield!

Four high yield summary points relating to the development of the diaphragm:

1. The muscles of the diaphragm are developed from the level of C3 to C5 (cervical somites 3, 4, and 5)
2. The septum transversum becomes the central tendon
3. The mesentery of the oesophagus makes up the crura of diaphragm and
4. The final position of the diaphragm is also determined by the growth of the lungs. As the lungs grow down, the diaphragm is also pushed in that direction.

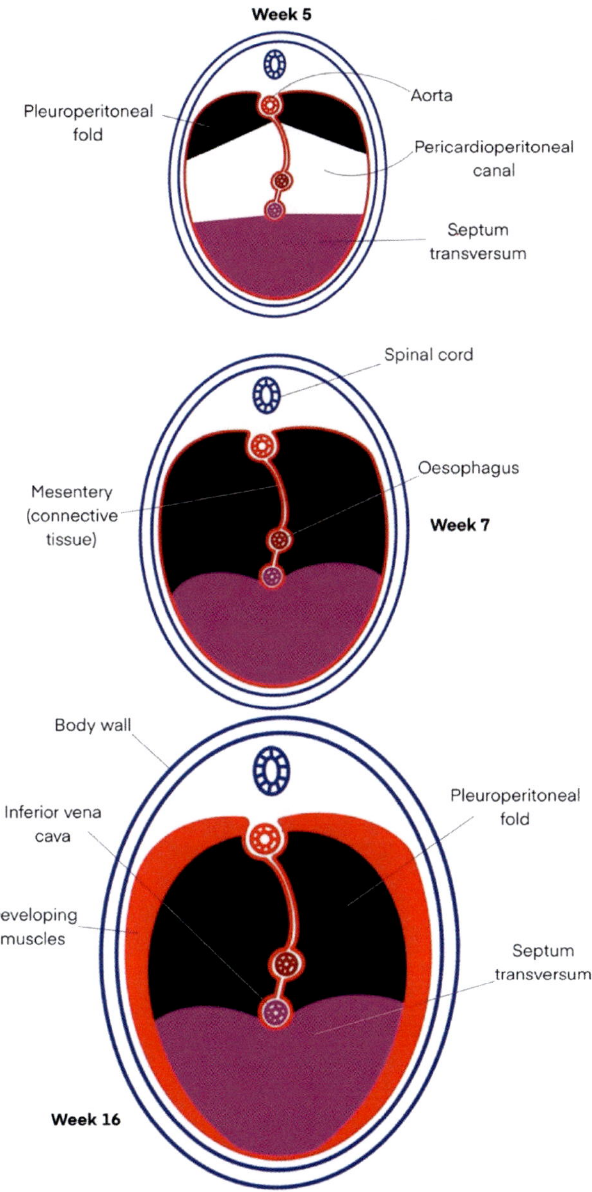

Image 13.1: Cross-sectional views of the diaphragm at various times demonstrating the progress of its development.

Chapter 14: The Bones

There isn't much to the embryology of the bones unless you want to learn about the molecular regulation. Chapter 14 will be relatively short. Essentially, the bones come from paraxial and parietal mesoderm as well as from the neural crest.

14.1 Endochondral bone formation

To simplify endochondral bone formation, here is a list of eight items in sequence of occurrence that summarise it. Use these eight dot-points with Image 14.1 to fully understand.

1. Undifferentiated tissue cells from the paraxial mesoderm turn into chondrocytes.
2. The chondrocytes form a template for the bone it is about to create.
3. Blood vessels enter this template right through the middle.
4. Osteoblasts enter the bone via this new highway of blood vessels.
5. The blood prevents chondrocytes growing towards the bone shaft.
6. Chondrocytes sacrifice their life following mineralisation of the template.
7. Osteoblasts take over the important role of depositing bone into the template, and the bone continues to grow for as long as osteoblasts allow them to do so at the growth plate.
8. When blood vessels enter the epiphyses, secondary ossification centres form.

14.2 The Skull

The neurocranium is your permanent helmet. The difference between the skull and the neurocranium is that the skull includes the bones of the face as well as the helmet, whereas the neurocranium consists of the flat bones and the cartilage that develops into the bones of the skull base (chondrocranium).

The flat bones come from the neural crest cells and the paraxial mesoderm which undergo ossification resulting in flat bone formation with spicules (Image 14.2). These spicules spread towards the outside covering almost the entire skull. In the newborn, the flat bones of the skull are separated by sutures and the areas that are not yet complete at this stage are called fontanelles.

The viscerocranium forms the bones of the face. They are formed by the first two pharyngeal arches (Chapter 9).

14.3 Vertebrae

The vertebrae come from somites (the paraxial mesoderm). Somite cells from both the left and the right paraxial mesoderm fuse together around the spinal cord and the notochord. Each vertebra is formed from the bottom half of one somite and the top half of the somite next to it. Mesenchymal cells fill the space between the vertebrae becoming the intervertebral disc. The notochord contributes to the intervertebral disc too.

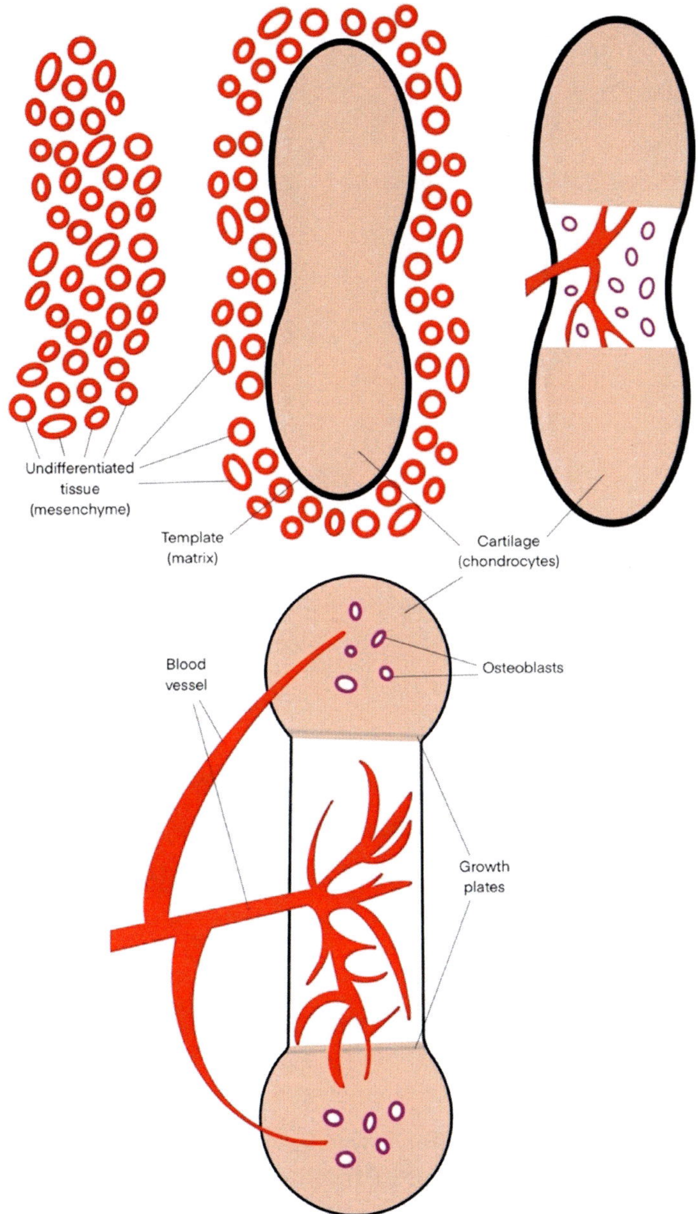

Image 14.1: Endochondral bone development.

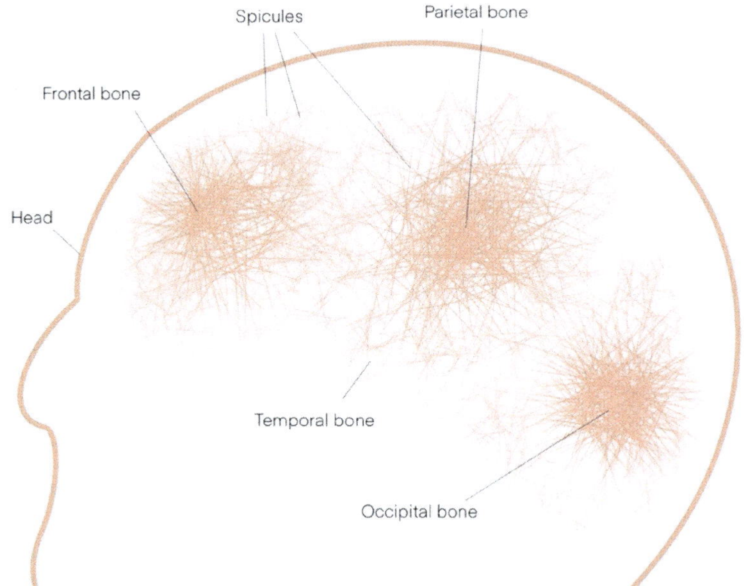

Image 14.2: Spicules spreading to form the neurocranium.

14.4 Ribs and sternum

The bony part of the ribs is derived from the sclerotome cells remaining in the paraxial mesoderm. They grow out from the thoracic vertebrae. The sternum develops from parietal lateral plate mesoderm.

14.5 The Limbs

By the end of the first month, limb buds grow out of the body. The buds are from the parietal mesoderm which forms the connective tissue and bones of limb and are covered by ectoderm (skin). The end of the limb forms hand plates and foot plates. Fingers and toes are finally formed when death of the cells between each finger and toe occurs. Joint cavities are also formed by cell death.

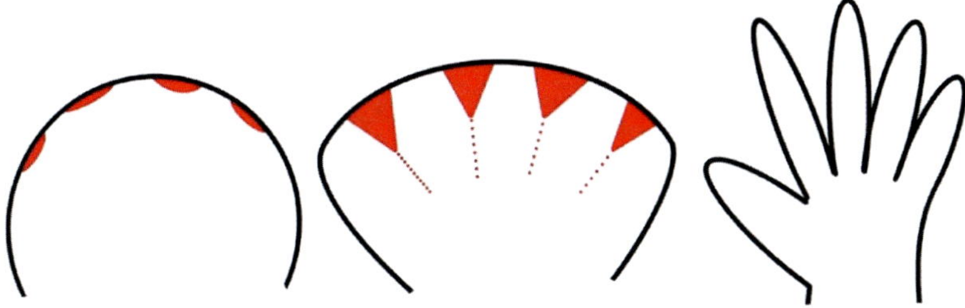

Image 14.3: Development of the distal limb in order from left to right. The areas in red indicate areas that are destroyed to form the fingers.

Chapter 15: The Skin

15.1 The Skin

The skin is made up of an epidermis and a dermis. The epidermis comes from ectoderm whereas the dermis comes from mesoderm. Neural crest cells (born from ectoderm) contribute to both layers.

In the beginning, the growing embryo is covered by ectoderm that is only a single layer of cells in thickness. However, these cells produce another layer of cells that completely cover the first layer. This process of differentiating and laying cells on top of each other is like building a brick house, and it continues until there are four layers. The basal layer is the layer that continually creates these new cells. The spinous layer lays directly above the basal layer. The granular layer is on top of the spinous layer, and the horny layer is the outermost layer. Keratin exists in the horny layer. This is a tough layer made from dead cells. From week 12 the neural crest cells enter the epidermis and are responsible for melanin synthesis from melanosomes. The dermis of the limbs and trunk are developed from lateral plate mesoderm. The paraxial mesoderm contributes to the dermis of the back. The neural crest cells form the dermis of the face and neck.

15.2 Hair

In some parts of the skin, parts of the basal layer that has invaded deeper into the dermis will form the hair buds. The mesoderm provides the hair with a blood supply. Some cells become keratinised forming the hair shaft. Surrounding the shaft is an epithelium layer called the hair sheath. Mesoderm helps form the dermal root sheath as well as to the arrector pili muscle. The hair grows by the ongoing multiplication of cells at the base of the hair shaft. The first hair that appears on the baby (lanugo) is lost at birth to make way for new follicles. Sebaceous glands are attached to the hair follicle and are created when epithelial cells of the hair bud enter the mesoderm.

15.3 The Sweat Glands

The sweat glands are formed from the epidermis (ectoderm) and they enter the dermis (mesoderm) and wind up. This is where sweat is produced. There are two types of sweat glands: eccrine and apocrine. Apocrine drain into the hair follicle, whereas the eccrine drain onto the surface of the skin. Sweat contains proteins, fats, and pheromones. The bad smell you sense when someone unhygienic walks past you in the supermarket is the result of bacteria breaking down these components of sweat.

If you have ever delivered a baby or watched a birth occur, you would notice that the baby is covered in a thick white paste. This is the vernix caseosa, which is secreted from the sebaceous glands to protect the baby from the amniotic fluid during its adventure in the womb. But now the baby is born, and their real adventure begins in life.

The end.